# The Ethics of Surveillance in Times of Emergency

# ENGAGING PHILOSOPHY

This series is a new forum for collective philosophical engagement with controversial issues in contemporary society.

**Disability in Practice**
*Attitudes, Policies, and Relationships*
Edited by Adam Cureton and Thomas E. Hill, Jr.

**Taxation**
*Philosophical Perspectives*
Edited by Martin O'Neill and Shepley Orr

**Bad Words**
*Philosophical Perspectives on Slurs*
Edited by David Sosa

**Academic Freedom**
Edited by Jennifer Lackey

**Lying**
*Language, Knowledge, Ethics, and Politics*
Edited by Eliot Michaelson and Andreas Stokke

**Treatment for Crime**
*Philosophical Essays on Neurointerventions in Criminal Justice*
Edited by David Birks and Thomas Douglas

**Games, Sports, and Play**
*Philosophical Essays*
Edited by Thomas Hurka

**Effective Altruism**
*Philosophical Issues*
Edited by Hilary Greaves and Theron Pummer

**Philosophy and Climate Change**
Edited by Mark Budolfson, Tristram McPherson, and David Plunkett

**Applied Epistemology**
Edited by Jennifer Lackey

**The Epistemology of Fake News**
Edited by Sven Bernecker, Amy K. Flowerree, and Thomas Grundmann

**The Ethics of Social Roles**
Edited by Alex Barber and Sean Cordell

# The Ethics of
# Surveillance in Times
# of Emergency

*Edited by*

KEVIN MACNISH AND ADAM HENSCHKE

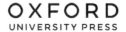

OXFORD
UNIVERSITY PRESS

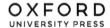

# OXFORD
UNIVERSITY PRESS

Great Clarendon Street, Oxford, OX2 6DP,
United Kingdom

Oxford University Press is a department of the University of Oxford.
It furthers the University's objective of excellence in research, scholarship,
and education by publishing worldwide. Oxford is a registered trade mark of
Oxford University Press in the UK and in certain other countries

Published in the United States of America by Oxford University Press
198 Madison Avenue, New York, NY 10016, United States of America

British Library Cataloguing in Publication Data
Data available

Library of Congress Control Number: 2023938527

ISBN 978-0-19-286491-8

DOI: 10.1093/oso/9780192864918.001.0001

Printed and bound in the UK by
Clays Ltd, Elcograf S.p.A.

Links to third party websites are provided by Oxford in good faith and
for information only. Oxford disclaims any responsibility for the materials
contained in any third party website referenced in this work.

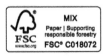

# Contents

## PART III ETHICS BY DESIGN IN SURVEILLANCE PROGRAMMES

# Acknowledgement

This work is part of the research programme Ethics of Socially Disruptive Technologies, which is funded through the Gravitation programme of the Dutch Ministry of Education, Culture, and Science and the Netherlands Organization for Scientific Research (NWO grant number 024.004.031)

# List of Contributors

**Haleh Asgarinia** is a PhD candidate at the University of Twente. Her PhD project involves the analysis of privacy issues in the context of large data set, AI-driven medical research. Her project is part of the Marie Skłodowska-Curie Innovative Training Network 'PROTECT—Protecting Personal Data Amidst Big Data Innovation', funded by the European Commission's Horizon 2020 programme, grant agreement No. 813497.

**Dr Katerina Hadjimatheou** is a Senior Lecturer in Criminology and Ethics at the University of Essex, UK. Her research focuses on the ethics of policing, of surveillance, and of big data and AI in a security context. She also works on the policing of violence against women and girls.

**Dr Adam Henschke** is an Assistant Professor with the Philosophy Section at the University of Twente. He works primarily in the ethics of technology, with much of his work focusing on security. He has written on the ethics of surveillance, the internet of things, human military enhancement, just war, counter-terrorism, and intelligence. Recent publications include the co-edited books *Counter-Terrorism, Ethics and Technology: Emerging Challenges at the Frontiers of Counter-Terrorism* (Springer), *The Palgrave Handbook of National Security* (Palgrave), and *Counter-Terrorism: The Ethical Issues* (Edward Elgar).

**Dr Katrina Hutchison** is a Senior Lecturer in the Department of Philosophy at Macquarie University. Her recent work has focused on issues of epistemic injustice, gender bias, and innovation. Katrina has been the recipient of an Australia Research Council 'Discovery Early Career Researcher Award', and was part of the development of the Macquarie Surgical Innovation Identification Tool (MSIIT) which has been used to inform policy on safely introducing surgical innovations.

**Dr Jane Johnson** is a field philosopher and Lecturer in the Department of Philosophy at Macquarie University. Her research focuses on questions in science and medicine, particularly around the ethics of emerging infectious diseases, animal ethics and epistemology, and the ethics of surgical innovation.

**Sahar Latheef** is a doctoral candidate in International, Political and Strategic Studies, at the Department of International Relations, Australian National University. Her research explores the ethical issues involved in using human enhancement applications in the military, focusing on cognitive enhancements and neurotechnology. Sahar has a background in biomedical engineering, neuroscience, and security studies. She has research experience in neuroscience focusing on cognitive disorders and currently works at the Department of Defence.

**Professor Kasper Lippert-Rasmussen** is Professor in Political Theory at University of Aarhus, Denmark, Professor II in Philosophy at University of Tromsø, Norway and Director of The Center for the Experimental-Philosophical Study of Discrimination. His main research interests are affirmative action, discrimination, equality, and ethics of blame. His most recent book is *The Beam and the Mote* (New York: Oxford University Press).

**Dr Björn Lundgren** is a postdoc at Utrecht University, working on a project on methodological issues raised by socially disruptive technologies. Lundgren has written about AI ethics, self-driving vehicles, privacy, anonymity, information, information security, decision under risk and uncertainty, and many other issues.

**Dr Kevin Macnish** is Head of Ethics Consulting at Sopra Steria Ltd. He was formerly Assistant Professor in ethics and technology at the University of Twente. He has published widely in ethics and surveillance, privacy and security. Recent books include *The Ethics of Surveillance: An Introduction* (Routledge, 2018) and, co-edited with Jai Galliott, *Big Data and Society* (Edinburgh University Press, 2020).

**Professor Seumas Miller** is Professor of Philosophy at the Australian Graduate School of Policing and Security at Charles Sturt University and Distinguished Research Fellow at the Uehiro Centre for Practical Ethics at the University of Oxford. He is the author of twenty-two books, including *The Ethics of Cybersecurity* (with T. Bossomaier) (Oxford University Press, 2023), and over 250 academic articles.

**Dr Kira Vrist Rønn** is Associate Professor at Department of Political Science and Public Management, University of Southern Denmark and Programme Director for the Master in Intelligence and Cyber Studies. Rønn's primary research interests are ethical issues related to policing, surveillance, and security studies.

**Dr Marcus Smith** is Associate Professor in Law at Charles Sturt University. He holds a PhD in law from the Australian National University. He has published widely on technology law and regulation. Recent books include: *Technology Law* (Cambridge University Press, 2021) and *Biometric Identification, Law and Ethics* (Springer, 2021).

**Dr Patrick Taylor Smith** is Resident Fellow at the Stockdale Center for Ethical Leadership at the United States Naval Academy. He was previously Assistant Professor of Philosophy at the University of Twente from 2018 to 2022, and Postdoctoral Fellow at the McCoy Center for Ethics in Society at Stanford University. He works primarily in social and political philosophy, with a special interest in the non-ideal application of neo-republican political theory to emerging technologies.

**Professor Tom Sorell** is Professor of Politics and Philosophy and Head of the Interdisciplinary Ethics Research Group at Warwick University. He was an RCUK Global Uncertainties Leadership Fellow (2013–2016). He was Tang Chun-I Visiting Professor in Philosophy at the Chinese University of Hong Kong in 2013. Previously, he was John Ferguson Professor of Global Ethics and Director of the Centre for the Study of Global Ethics, University of Birmingham.

**Dr Frej Klem Thomsen** is Chief Consultant with the Danish Dataethics Council at the Danish National Centre for Ethics in in Copenhagen, Denmark. He specializes in criminal justice ethics, the ethics of discrimination, surveillance ethics, and data ethics.

# Introduction

*Kevin Macnish and Adam Henschke*

The appearance of Covid-19, and the declaration by the WHO of its status as a pandemic, led to the most widespread institution of states of emergency around the globe in history (Adhanom 2020; Greene 2020). Most governments instituted some form of lockdown, suspending businesses and all but essential travel. As the lockdowns lifted, with a view to restarting the global economy, states engaged in large-scale surveillance to track and trace the spread of the virus (Tsang 2020; Gershgorn 2020). These efforts predominantly focused on technological solutions, usually in the form of applications to be hosted on citizens' smart phones. The advantage with such solutions being that they could cope with the large volumes of people involved, crunch the data quickly and effectively to keep abreast of the spread of the virus in country, and alert users to the possibility that they had contracted the virus.

Whatever the efficacy of such applications, and this has been questioned (Soltani, Calo, and Bergstrom 2020), the proposal and institution of such widespread surveillance raises serious ethical issues. This is particularly true for liberal democracies, in which individual freedoms, including the human right of non-absolute privacy, are particularly important. Within this liberal democratic context, the ethical analysis of surveillance has generally focused, for obvious reasons, on state and corporate surveillance of individuals and groups in society (surveillance as control). This has for the most part been critical, with an emphasis placed on resistance to exercises of power (Bakir 2015; Gilliom 2001; Marx 2003). Despite this focus, some have considered the ethics of surveillance as care (Lyon 2007; Stoddart 2012), while others have attempted to seek balance in state and corporate acts of surveillance over the more critical approaches (Macnish 2014; Marx 1998; A. L. Allen 2008; Henschke 2017).

The appearance and rapid global transmission of Covid-19 in 2019–20 therefore led to a shift of emphasis, for some at least, from surveillance as control to surveillance as care. The obvious healthcare implications of a virus which threatened to overwhelm national health systems and killed over a million people were such that surveillance became seen as more acceptable, or even a duty of governments when it came to protecting their citizens.

Kevin Macnish and Adam Henschke, *Introduction* In: *The Ethics of Surveillance in Times of Emergency.*
Edited by: Kevin Macnish and Adam Henschke, Oxford University Press. © Oxford University Press 2023.
DOI: 10.1093/oso/9780192864918.003.0001

At the heart of these issues is the question of the relationship between the individual and the state in a liberal democracy during states of emergency (Agamben 2005). During wartime, it is often accepted that certain civil liberties (and even some human rights) should be put on hold for the duration of the war to aid the state in protecting its citizens (Walzer 2015; Bellamy 2008). However, and despite the political rhetoric in some quarters, while a response to a virus may in some ways resemble a war, there are significant differences between fighting people and 'fighting' a virus. People have intentions while viruses do not; people, unlike viruses, respond to rumour and intelligence; and the distribution and nature of the harms of war, particularly when fought on or over domestic soil, are distinct from those of a virus. This raises questions about legitimate levels of secrecy and transparency when it comes to state responses to the occasioning crisis.

This is not to say that states of emergency are not appropriate in response to pandemics. Rather, it is to add nuance to the temptation to engage extreme and unjustified responses. It is overly simplistic to draw on historical wartime analogies to see what is appropriate. Furthermore, the history of citizens' relationship with their governments has changed since any large-scale states of emergency were declared, at least in the global North (Waldron 2003; Sagar 2007). Trust in government has declined significantly since 1945, for instance, and particularly so in the wake of the MPs expense scandal in the UK, the polarization of politics in the US, and 9/11 and the subsequent Snowden revelations. Function creep of government powers is a related, widely recognized problem, with special powers given to the US government in the wake of 9/11 remaining in place despite the demise of the original enemy against whom they were instituted (Philips 1984; Rijt 2011).

Furthermore, even in states of emergency, liberal democracies have sought to distance themselves from authoritarian states by stressing the voluntary nature of the proposed surveillance. Yet the proposed track and trace applications were originally estimated to require adoption by 60 per cent of the population to be successful (Clarke 2020). Given that, it is not clear how such an adoption rate can be guaranteed in the absence of coercion, especially given the decline in trust of governments. Without this level of adoption, should the technology be abandoned or continue to monitor the activities of a few virtuous adoptees even while it has no chance of success, at least according to its original terms? Alternatively, should liberal democratic governments abandon the principle of consent in this issue and follow authoritarian regimes in coercing adoption?

It may be that privacy is a minor value to sacrifice in the aim of saving lives. Furthermore, the track and trace technology will not (always) collect information relating to conversations, or even (necessarily) location data, hence protecting users' privacy to some degree. Nonetheless, locational privacy remains a concern, and many of the proposed applications could be used to identify gatherings of individuals (and potentially identify those individuals) which would be of interest to governments for other reasons, such as tracking activists or groups of 'undesirables'. Locational privacy is in the public interest as well as the health of the nation and needs to be balanced against public health concerns more carefully than through mere appeals to 'if you have done nothing wrong, you will have nothing to hide' (Macnish 2018; Solove 2007).

It may also be that digital divides in society deepen because of the technology used. Access to smart phones is not universal, with some struggling to afford these phones and others lacking the mental competence or dexterity to use them (Himma 2007; Abbey and Hyde 2009). In such cases, further technical solutions have been proposed, such as smart cards or wearables, that would still monitor the person's whereabouts without requiring a smart phone. Even here, though, the Collingridge dilemma holds, whereby we cannot know all the societal impacts of new technologies until those technologies have been implemented, and by then it is often too late to reverse those impacts (Collingridge 1982). Such impacts could include public–private lock-in, whereby governments using technologies designed by corporations become reliant on those technologies, and hence those corporations; and normalization of surveillance in society such that most will accept heightened levels of surveillance continuing after the emergency has receded.

These are by no means all the ethical issues raised by the current appeal to technological responses to the Covid-19 pandemic, but they are sufficient to establish the importance of ethical reflection. Beyond this, many of these issues will apply for other states of emergency, be they caused by viruses, humans, or natural disasters. The Covid-19 pandemic, and the proposed response, therefore provides a powerful impetus to ask when, and to what extent, surveillance can be justified during states of emergency.

This book hence draws from the use of surveillance technologies introduced during the Covid-19 pandemic to explore a set of issues and challenges facing decision makers and designers in times of emergency: how do we respond to emergencies in ways that are both consistent with democratic and community principles, and that are ethically justifiable? Emergencies like public health pandemics not only place stress on existing infrastructure and communities but put significant pressure on our decision-making. While an unsophisticated consequentialism will simply suggest that we choose the option that saves the most lives or favours some other large-scale good outcome, the political, ethical, and practical realities are, as already noted, far more complex and require much greater nuance. The use of surveillance technologies during public health crises is a vital frame to explore the challenge of acting in times of emergency. Moreover, as an exercise in reflective applied ethics, the chapters do not just seek to apply a given theory or principle to the problem of surveillance in times of emergency but use the challenges facing us to critically engage with, reflect upon, and develop those theories and principles.

The book's authors recognize this challenge—is it possible to respond to exceptional conditions in ways that preserve our core values, or must these core values be subsumed under the need to respond to the particular emergency? On the one hand, the pluralism that is threaded through liberal democracies, and even many modern non-liberal democratic nations, holds that we take multiple values seriously. On the other hand, as we have seen with the Covid-19 pandemic, to fulfil their responsibility to keep people safe, governments every-where have engaged in a range of policies, practices, and applications of existing technologies that would have been impermissible in normal circumstances. The book offers responses to this challenge by looking at three interrelated ways that that challenge can manifest: first, the democratic challenges; second, the ethical challenges; and third the design challenges faced in developing ethical solutions.

## Democracy in Times of Emergency

Part I looks at the ways that democratic values are placed under stress in times of emergency. Liberal democracies generally hold to a set of values that see the individual as having priority in how decisions ought to be made, but when there are large numbers of lives at stake, and time is limited, decision makers must find ways to protect the lives and liberties of their people, whilst retaining that which makes liberal democracies what they are. This first section of the book places the global pandemic in a context of political responsibility: what must decision makers do, and how does this square with their commitment to liberal democratic values? Surveillance is a useful way to frame these core political challenges as it places the need for the state to have oversight of what is happening, in tension with basic principles like privacy and free movement. As is so often the case, such extreme conditions that call for increased surveillance can shed significant light on democratic ideals, theories, and practices.

Tom Sorrell's chapter sets the scene by looking at how emergencies and surveillance threaten basic notions of liberty and freedom in democracies but argues that such threats may be justified. He holds that pandemic surveillance should not be seen as one *more* instance of centralized state surveillance of populations, as if it were an intensification of a single trend started with bulk collection by the NSA and GCHQ for counter-terrorist purposes. On the contrary, he claims, in some of its intense forms it is strongly disanalogous morally to bulk collection and its associated data analytics for preventing terrorist attacks. Rather, pandemic surveillance is open to a strong moral justification, tied to the status of virology and epidemiology as sciences, and the strong independent justifiability of public health measures, including those that temporarily restrict liberty. Isolation and electronic surveillance for contact tracing may arguably save many more lives and prevent much more harm than network analysis by the intelligence services, as the quick flattening of death rates in high-surveillance jurisdictions shows when compared to exponential rises in other countries, and when surveillance effects along these lines are compared with credible estimates of numbers of lives saved by counter-terrorism. Hence the ethics of surveillance during pandemics is not primarily to be judged by privacy considerations, but by its connections to sufficiently inclusive, properly timed, and accurate tests of the presence of the virus. When a testing regime is inadequate, the intrusiveness or privacy protection of the associated electronic surveillance is of secondary importance morally.

Patrick Taylor Smith uses a neo-republican approach to argue that in times of emergency, such as a pandemic, democracies might be permitted to enter a form of limited dictatorship. His chapter makes three related points. First, he offers an account of emergency that is normatively relevant: an emergency occurs when there is a rapid shift in the relative risks of private and public domination that disrupts an existing institutional equilibrium. Second, he argues that—contrary to standard views—we should understand that institutions cannot change instantly and that emergencies should not be understood as justifying a permissively consequentialist political morality. Rather, using the Roman concept of 'dictator' as example, he holds that neo-republicans should create regulated spaces for controlled emergency reasoning. That is, like special prosecutors or inspectors general, the idea is to create institutions that make it possible for nimble policy reactions that are nonetheless constrained in scope, duration, and resources. This creates a set of checks on those actors. Finally, he applies this account to the question of surveillance in the case of serious global health emergencies.

Seumas Miller and Marcus Smith look at the collective responsibility for citizens to engage in surveillance processes like track and trace. As already noted, strategies for combating Covid-19 involve a complex set of often compet-ing, and sometimes interconnected (e.g., some privacy rights, such as control over personal data, are themselves aspects of autonomy) moral considerations, and so hard choices must be made. However, the idea of a collective responsibility on the part of individuals to jointly suffer some costs, e.g., loss of privacy rights, in favour of a collective good (eliminating or containing the spread of Covid-19) lies at the heart of all such effective strategies. This idea provides the theoretical framework for their chapter. Accordingly, they provide an analysis of the appropriate notion of collective responsibility. This theoretical framework is applied to a variety of surveillance tools, including phone metadata tracking, used to combat Covid-19. However, in doing so the wider context of the so-called 'surveillance society' is considered, as are a range of potentially competing collective goods, i.e., not merely aggregate loss of life because of the pandemic.

Haleh Asgarinia takes a different angle in considering the placing of groups under surveillance. She notes that, to control outbreaks of disease, quarantine decisions may be taken based on tracking the transmission of the disease on the group level. However, targeting groups as potential carriers of a disease, rather than addressing individuals as patients, gives rise to questions regarding the privacy of groups. In such cases, the cluster-type groupings designed by data analytics are sources of information for making policy decisions without focusing on individual identifiability. Since privacy concerns on the individual level arise when individuals are made identifiable, groups designed by algorithms or models may expose the crowd to privacy harms which they would not otherwise experience. At the same time, obligations or regulations developed to protect individuals from the misuse of their data are not helpful at the level of the group. Furthermore, data protection rules cannot protect groups against possible privacy harms because many of the uses of data that involve algorithmic groupings are used for the purpose of scientific research and improving public health. These suggest that while there are rules and obligations for privacy and data protection at the level of the individual, there is a growing need to protect groups as entities. This requires a deeper examination of group privacy and how the privacy of the group is considered in the context of data protection.

In a similar manner, Katrina Hutchison and Jane Johnson argue in their chapter that the type of knowledge aimed at by surveillance may differ from that derived from other kinds of knowledge. Hence people diagnosed with Covid-19 give contact tracers a different kind of knowledge from technologically derived data such as that from a phone's GPS or more socially mandated and technologically mediated data generated from a phone app's sign-in data. Having outlined these differences, they look at some of the ethical dimensions that arise from the ways that this knowledge is generated and used, particularly looking at the risks of epistemic injustice.

## Ethics in Times of Emergency

Part II looks at particular ethical challenges faced in times of emergency. The use of surveillance technologies, and their impact on basic freedoms, are not only of political importance but speak to deeper ethical discussions around the very nature of what one can and should do in emergencies. By looking at the ways that different surveillance technologies have been used to respond to Covid-19, we are forced to consider whom we hold responsible, for how long, and what rights can be justifiably limited?

Kasper Lippert-Rasmussen and Kira Vrist Rønn open Part II by drawing from recent discussions in the just war tradition to explore the relations between the liability for risks that an individual poses to others in times of pandemics with the notion of informed consent and surveillance. They note that, in the case of pandemics at least, there is no human *aggressor* and thus the antagonistic relationship between *the surveillant* and *the surveilled*, which is commonly assumed to obtain in much of the literature on surveillance ethics, does not exist in this context. Yet many scholars have drawn on distinctions from just war theory to develop a framework for surveillance ethics which focus on considerations regarding the *liability* of the surveilled and how it affects the moral permissibility of surveillance. In their chapter they address the question of whether and in what form liability should play a role in surveillance ethics in the context of pandemics. Here they identify the dilemma between the developers and health authorities in many countries, emphasizing that *voluntariness* on the side of the users of these apps are key attributes and the need for widespread use of the app to obtain the desired effect. However, such levels of usage are unlikely to be achieved if voluntariness is respected. This provides an opportunity to explore the role of voluntariness in non-antagonistic surveillance ethics.

Sahar Latheef also considers voluntariness through the lens of informed consent, and how public surveillance may lead to trade-offs in this context. She assesses the salient features of track and trace apps to determine whether these introduce novel concerns regarding informed consent and individual rights, particularly in the case of features which allow apps to identify and communicate with other proximate devices. In this case, she holds, an individual is consenting to allow access to their information and, to some extent at least, to the access of information of other people within a specific proximity. This leads to a consideration of inter-agency data sharing and how the data collected could be used for purposes other than contact tracing (for example in criminal investigations). As such, the chapter provides an understanding of the necessary trade-offs made with regards to individual rights to informed consent to achieve a vital public health goal.

Katerina Hadjimatheou considers how surveillance should be used to police protest during emergencies. Following announcements by police in England and Wales to intensify surveillance, using informants and undercover police, against groups protesting climate change, Hadjimatheou uses this relationship as her case study. As with Asgarinia, she notes that the nature of these groups mean that they cannot be reduced to aggregate exercises of individuals' rights, and so such a study must look at the impact of surveillance on the groups themselves. In this, she considers two angles: the first is the impact of covert human surveillance (aka undercover policing), while the second is the conceptualization of that impact through developing the notion of 'chill'. While chilling effects are often referenced (Macnish 2015; Columbia Law Review 1969; Kaminski and Witnov 2015) they are rarely evidenced, with some notable exceptions (PEN International 2014). This chapter addresses that lack. Based on this evidence, she argues that the impact of chilling effects needs to be understood at the group level as well as the individual. As such, chilling effects arising from surveillance can be detrimental to those under surveillance, particularly protestors, and those who may benefit from their protests in a democratic environment.

Adam Henschke then looks at the need to ensure that ethical norms return to pre-emergency conditions. He argues that situations such as public health emergencies rely on a dynamic ethics and, as such, consideration must be given on how to reverse social norms that arise during these emergencies. First, on a dynamic view, emergencies, and the exceptional justifications arising through such emergencies, do come to an end. While a great deal of ethical discussion looks at the conditions about when an 'emergency ethics' becomes operational, much less has been said about the end period. Second, picking up from the importance of what happens when an emergency ends, while certain policies and practices might be justifiable in response to the Covid-19 pandemic, he holds there is a need to ensure that such policies are reversed once the emergency has receded, and that the social norms around particular surveillance practices and policies return to pre-emergency state. This is especially the case when considering the surveillance policies and technologies that were introduced during the Covid-19 pandemic. While many other emergency policies are obviously and persistently intrusive, many of the surveillance policies and technologies that were introduced during the Covid-19 emergency were subtle, invisible, and pervasive. This means that the social norms around surveillance are less likely to return to pre-emergency norms and as such, the surveillance practices during the emergency have a significant capacity not only to persist once the emergency ends but to influence and drive other social norms around surveillance. Given these points, he argues that the surveillance policies and technologies introduced during the Covid-19 pandemic show that emergency surveillance ought to be considered as justifiable but abnormal and he gives suggestions on how to ensure that the surveillance justified by public health ethics remains abnormal.

## Ethics by Design in Surveillance Programmes

The final part of the book closes off by looking at the ways that ethical principles can help design surveillance programmes, and aid in decision-making in times of emergency more generally. A foundational ethical principle, proportionality, is frequently drawn upon to justify particular responses. At its simplest, proportionality is a very useful and intuitive principle—in seeking to respond to an emergency, how significant are the impacts of the emergency, and what are the effects of different responses. Again, with regard to surveillance technologies and practices, we can see the pivotal role that proportionality plays in emergency situations. Moreover, the contributions in this section use surveillance technologies to shed light on the concept of proportionality, and the ways that this principle is designed into technologies.

Lundgren begins this final part of the book with an exploration of the practicality of questions that have been proposed to ensure well designed pandemic surveillance programmes, and that such a programme should be rolled out globally, while also providing a set of ethical guidelines for contact tracing apps. Like Henschke, he argues that emergency surveillance must be temporary. Yet temporary laws can become permanent, even with so-called sunset clauses. Moreover, temporary measures that are widely adapted can change norms, such as the speed with which social media has changed many people's norms of information distribution. Thus, even temporary usage of emergency surveillance can have permanent effects. It is also important to ask what effects increased surveillance in a democratic society will have on surveillance in non-democratic societies. For example, President Trump's behaviour and rhetoric about 'fake news' have been used by oppressive regimes and there is, similarly, a risk that emergency surveillance in liberal democracies can influence the ability of oppressive regimes to use and abuse surveillance free from challenge.

Frej Klem Thomsen looks at the role that the principle of proportionality plays in morally permissible surveillance. He argues that the only difference between states of emergency and ordinary circumstances is that the stakes are greater in a state of emergency. This entails that an account of morally permissible surveillance should be unexceptional: there is no clear-cut separation between ordinary circumstances and emergencies, but rather a spectrum between them (Statman 2012). He then sketches an *unexceptional* theory of permissible surveillance in *exceptional* circumstances, offering definitions of key principles and discussing certain features of particular interest. He too recognizes that an important risk for the use of surveillance to support the containment of pandemics is the danger of function creep or normalization of the exception, where practices of surveillance that are permissible during the emergency are sustained after the return to ordinary circumstances. In response, he argues that the situation with respect to this risk is likely tragic: the situations in which there is a genuine risk are also those situations in which state agents are most likely to pursue surveillance regardless of the risk.

Finally, Kevin Macnish sheds light on further challenges around proportionality by asking if we are too focussed on technological fixes to things like pandemics, overlooking non-technological options in our proportionality calculations. Consistent with this part of the book, he begins with a discussion of proportionality, which demonstrates that there are different ways of understanding and using the term, which in turn leads to confusion in the public debate. He then examines how the technology used in emergency surveillance, in trying to square the liberal democratic circles of privacy and surveillance as well as voluntariness and a need for high adoption, may lead to false positive and false negatives. These come together to demonstrate that technology may be seen as proportionate in the light of one approach and yet disproportionate in the light of alternative approaches. He suggests that these alternatives are often not presented to the public debate owing to a tendency towards techno-fetishism, a default assumption in favour of technical fixes over non-technical alternatives. He concludes that the form of surveillance undertaken by many such technical fixes, careful as they may be, may nonetheless be disproportionate responses to the crises they seek to address.

# References

Abbey, Ruth, and Sarah Hyde. 2009. 'No Country for Older People? Age and the Digital Divide'. *Journal of Information, Communication and Ethics in Society* 7 (4): 225–42. https://doi.org/10.1108/14779960911004480.

Adam, Henschke. 2018. 'Are The Costs Of Metadata Worth It? Conceptualising Proportionality And Its Relation To Metadata'. In *Intelligence and the Function of Government*, edited by Daniel Baldino and Rhys Crawley. Melbourne University Press.

Adhanom, Tedros. 2020. 'WHO Director-General's Opening Remarks at the Media Briefing on COVID-19 - 11 March 2020'. 11 March 2020. https://www.who.int/dg/speeches/detail/who-director-general-s-opening-remarks-at-the-media-briefing-on-covid-19—11-march-2020.

Agamben, Giorgio. 2005. *State of Exception*. Chicago: University of Chicago Press.

Allen, Anita L. 2008. 'The Virtuous Spy: Privacy as an Ethical Limit'. *The Monist* 91 (1): 3–22.

Bakir, Viand. 2015. '"Veillant Panoptic Assemblage": Mutual Watching and Resistance to Mass Surveillance after Snowden'. *Media and Communication* 3 (3): 12–25.

Bellamy, Alex J. 2008. 'The Ethics of Terror Bombing: Beyond Supreme Emergency'. *Journal of Military Ethics* 7 (1): 41–65. https://doi.org/10.1080/15027570801953448.

Clarke, Laurie. 2020. 'How Will the NHS Covid-19 Contact Tracing App Work and When Will It Go Live?' *NS Tech* (blog). 5 May 2020. https://tech.newstatesman.com/security/nhs-covid-19-contact-tracing-app-rollout.

Collingridge, David. 1982. *Social Control of Technology*. London: Continuum International Publishing Group Ltd.

Columbia Law Review. 1969. 'The Chilling Effect in Constitutional Law'. *Columbia Law Review* 69 (5): 808–42.

Gershgorn, Dave. 2020. 'We Mapped How the Coronavirus Is Driving New Surveillance Programs Around the World'. Medium. 19 May 2020. https://onezero.medium.com/the-pandemic-is-a-trojan-horse-for-surveillance-programs-around-the-world-887fa6f12ec9.

Gilliom, John. 2001. *Overseers of the Poor: Surveillance, Resistance, And The Limits Of Privacy*. 1 edition. Chicago: University of Chicago Press.

Greene, Alan. 2020. 'State of Emergency: How Different Countries Are Invoking Extra Powers to Stop the Coronavirus'. The Conversation. 30 March 2020. http://theconversation.com/state-of-emergency-how-different-countries-are-invoking-extra-powers-to-stop-the-coronavirus-134495.

Henschke, Adam. 2017. *Ethics in an Age of Surveillance: Personal Information and Virtual Identities*. New York: Cambridge University Press.

Himma, Kenneth Einar. 2007. 'The Information Gap, the Digital Divide, and the Obligations of Affluent Nations'. *International Review of Information Ethics* 7 (9): 3–4.

Kaminski, Margot E., and Shane Witnov. 2015. 'The Conforming Effect: First Amendment Implications of Surveillance, Beyond Chilling Speech'. SSRN Scholarly Paper ID 2550385. Rochester, NY: Social Science Research Network. http://papers.ssrn.com/abstract=2550385.

Lyon, David. 2007. *Surveillance Studies: An Overview*. 1 edition. Cambridge, UK; Malden, MA: Polity Press.

Macnish, Kevin. 2014. 'Just Surveillance? Towards a Normative Theory of Surveillance'. *Surveillance and Society* 12 (1): 142–53.

Macnish, Kevin. 2015. 'An Eye for an Eye: Proportionality and Surveillance'. *Ethical Theory and Moral Practice* 18 (3): 529–48. https://doi.org/10.1007/s10677-014-9537-5.

Macnish, Kevin. 2018. *The Ethics of Surveillance: An Introduction*. 1 edition. London : New York: Routledge.

Marx, Gary T. 1998. 'Ethics for the New Surveillance'. *The Information Society* 14: 171–85.

Marx, Gary T. 2003. 'A Tack in the Shoe: Neutralizing and Resisting the New Surveillance'. *Journal of Social Issues* 59 (2): 369–90. https://doi.org/10.1111/1540-4560.00069.

PEN International. 2014. 'Global Chilling: The Impact of Mass Surveillance on International Writers'. PEN American Center.

Philips, Michael. 1984. 'Are Coerced Agreements Involuntary?' *Law and Philosophy* 3 (1): 133–45. https://doi.org/10.1007/BF00211227.

Rijt, Jan-Willem van der. 2011. 'Coercive Interference and Moral Judgment'. *Ethical Theory and Moral Practice* 14 (5): 549–67. https://doi.org/10.1007/s10677-011-9262-2.

Sagar, Rahul. 2007. 'On Combating the Abuse of State Secrecy*'. *Journal of Political Philosophy* 15 (4): 404–27. https://doi.org/10.1111/j.1467-9760.2007.00283.x.

Solove, Daniel J. 2007. '"I've Got Nothing to Hide" and Other Misunderstandings of Privacy'. *San Diego Law Review* 44: 745–72.

Soltani, Ashkan, Ryan Calo, and Carl Bergstrom. 2020. 'Contact-Tracing Apps Are Not a Solution to the COVID-19 Crisis'. *Brookings* (blog). 27 April 2020. https://www.brookings.edu/techstream/inaccurate-and-insecure-why-contact-tracing-apps-could-be-a-disaster/.

Statman, D. 2012. 'Supreme Emergencies and the Continuum Problem'. Journal of Military Ethics 11 (4): 287–98.

Stoddart, Eric. 2012. 'A Surveillance of Care'. In *Routledge Handbook of Surveillance Studies*, edited by Kirstie Ball, Kevin Haggerty, and David Lyon, 369–76. Abingdon, Oxon; New York: Routledge.

Tsang, Samantha. 2020. 'Here Are the Contact Tracing Apps Being Deployed around the World'. 28 April 2020. https://iapp.org/news/a/here-are-the-contact-tracing-apps-being-employed-around-the-world/.

Waldron, Jeremy. 2003. 'Security and Liberty: The Image of Balance'. *Journal of Political Philosophy* 11 (2): 191–210. https://doi.org/10.1111/1467-9760.00174.

Walzer, Michael. 2015. *Just and Unjust Wars: A Moral Argument with Historical Illustrations*. 5th ed. Basic Books.

# PART I
# DEMOCRACY IN TIMES OF EMERGENCY

# 1

# Pandemic Population Surveillance

## Privacy and Life-Saving

*Tom Sorell*

In an interview with Vice TV on 12 April 2020, Edward Snowden claimed that the technology that was being developed and applied in the West for reporting Covid symptoms and for tracing contacts was part of an 'architecture of oppression' (Dowd 2020). Snowden rose to prominence in 2013 after exposing large-scale data mining operations by the U.S. National Security Agency (NSA). The NSA had, among other things, investigated patterns of telephone communication between terrorist suspects, or their known associates, and other, up to then unnoticed, telephone users. Some of the latter became targets for further investigation.

Snowden's remarks in the April interview clearly suggested that Covid surveillance was one *more* example of surveillance by Western states on their own populations, an example to be added to programmes of counter-terrorist surveillance on the part of the American NSA and British GCHQ that Snowden exposed in 2013. While conceding that symptom tracking and tracing was prima facie beneficial, Snowden said that the data gathered would be retained after the pandemic and might well be used somehow against citizens.

This paper rejects Snowden's claims. I argue that pandemic surveillance in many Western countries, including the UK, is *nothing like* NSA and GCHQ collection and mining of communications data. It is carried out by very different agents, for very different purposes, on the basis of much more reliable evidence of an imminent and genuine threat to life. It is very far from being *secret* surveillance, and the technology used is very different from bulk collection technology. In jurisdictions in which it was carried out soon enough after the Covid epidemic began to spread from Wuhan, probably in November or December 2019, surveillance saved many more thousands of lives than the NSA or GCHQ surveillance has. Its record of life-saving amply justifies it on balance, even when it has been unnecessarily intrusive.

The rest of this paper is organized as follows. I first consider how public health pandemic surveillance is supposed to operate in the early stages of a virus outbreak. Up to a point, this type of response was implemented by East Asian jurisdictions, notably South Korea, using high tech data collection, fusion of datasets, and analytics. These methods of surveillance operated in the context of

Tom Sorell, *Pandemic Population Surveillance: Privacy and Life-Saving* In: *The Ethics of Surveillance in Times of Emergency*. Edited by: Kevin Macnish and Adam Henschke, Oxford University Press. © Oxford University Press 2023. DOI: 10.1093/oso/9780192864918.003.0002 quick, comprehensive, and effective testing for the virus. The approach was successful at flattening the rate of local infection and consequently preventing large numbers of deaths from the disease. In South Korea, the epidemic was not only contained and contained quickly, but the lockdowns experienced in many countries in the rest of the world were avoided, along with their economic costs.

In the second section I turn to test, track, and trace in the UK. The UK was *not* able to contain the first wave of the virus but succeeded in reducing its spread and lives lost after a very widespread lockdown of local travel and economic activity. It was only after the lockdown succeeded that testing at the right scale and at the right speed started to become generally available. After September 2020, test, track and trace slowed down or was unavailable in the right places and on the right scale to meet demand. Electronic contact tracing, which was supposed to operate in tandem with symptom reporting, was slow to be developed, late to be made available to the public, and, I shall argue, disproportionately concerned with privacy protection.

I come in section three to Snowden's claim that electronic contact tracing contributes to an architecture of oppression. Not only is this highly dubious in the light of the widely accepted privacy concerns of UK tracing app developers and their Western European counterparts; it does not even seem to apply to the approach of South Korea. Although the South Koreans did make use of bulk datasets, and some of the same analytics as have been used by Western intelligence services against counter-terrorism, the connection between using those techniques and saving large numbers of lives is much better evidenced and scientifically understood in the case of Covid than in the case of post-9/11 terrorism. Again, although South Korea's infection notifications were sometimes unduly privacy-violating, this does not outweigh or undercut the moral value of its general approach to containment.

## The Case of South Korea

Pandemic response is time sensitive. The World Health Organization (WHO) recognizes six phases of a pandemic, followed by a post-peak period and a post-pandemic period (WHO 2020a). Phase 1 is the period during which a virus spreads between animals only. Phase 2 is in many ways the most crucial. It occurs when animal-to-human transmission is first observed, and when a test, track, and isolate system is applied to identify and place out of circulation those who are infected. It is effective action at Phase 2 that pre-empts the sort of disruptive and economically damaging counter-measures implemented after March 2020 in the UK.

The official WHO timeline for Covid begins on 31 December 2019 (WHO 2021b), but it is based on an official communication from the local Wuhan public health authorities based on earlier observed 'viral pneumonia'—probably misclassified Covid. How much earlier than late December this 'viral pneumonia' was reported is unclear, but let us suppose that animal to human transmission of what was in fact the new corona virus started in or near Wuhan in November 2019 or slightly earlier. Then there was probably a short period in which a lockdown at its point of origin and strongly enforced transport prohibitions would have kept the pandemic in Wuhan in Phase 2. When that was no longer possible, containment in the places to which it spread next might have succeeded. Containment did succeed in some places relatively close to Wuhan: Taiwan, for example, and South Korea. It did not succeed in many places connected to China by air travel: Italy and the United Kingdom are notable cases in point.

The WHO strategy for Covid response, then, aimed at first at the *containment* of the virus. This involved notification of symptoms by individuals to doctors and public health authorities. Close to the beginning of the outbreak, the list of recognized symptoms was less specific—a continuous cough and a temperature— than it has become since. After notification, those with symptoms were to be given quick antigen testing. If the test was positive, the infected person was to self-isolate or submit to externally supervised quarantine. Contacts of those testing positive were then to be traced. In East Asian countries with experience of the earlier SARS epidemic, high-tech contact tracing was used, and some of it was highly intrusive.

The first case of Covid in South Korea (I base my account in this paragraph on Dighe et al. 2020; see also Kennedy 2020) was reported on 20 January 2020. The initial half-dozen cases all had a connection with Wuhan or Hubei province in China. In about a month, the number of cases had risen to around thirty, with some infections also imported from Japan, Thailand and Singapore. The thirty-first case, recorded on 18 February, became notorious for being associated with a 'super-spreader' in the South Korean city of Daegu, who had visited Wuhan. She was affiliated with a religious organization called Shincheongi, and participated in close-contact religious rituals with other members of the group. On 20 February, seventy new cases were reported, and testing among members of Shincheongi revealed 544 cases of the infection out of 4400 tested. By 29 February, however, the peak daily infection number (990) was reached in South Korea. This declined to 131 on 10 March, and 47 on 6 April.

South Korea, then, managed an impressively rapid containment. How? Briefly, by intense virus testing and by quick and effective contact tracing for those testing positive or reporting symptoms (A timeline of actions can be found at Cha and Kim 2020). South Korean contact tracing involved not just consulting the infected person's memory of contacts and places visited, but also tracking using CCTV from ATM and credit card transactions (Roth 2020), or mobile phone tracking using location data from cell towers. Mobile phones identified in the neighbour-hood of an infected person's recent location history were then sent messages notifying them of possible contact with a virus carrier and inviting phone owners for tests. Occasionally, the communications to neighbourhoods contained identifying, even intimate, information about the relevant spreader of the virus, creating conditions for stigmatization or, even worse, possible retaliation. For example, visits to 'love hotels' were included in public location histories of spreaders, and communicated to possible contacts (Zastrow 2020).

The South Korean approach to Covid track and trace departed from more than one norm of privacy protection in normal times. First, probably without democratic deliberation, it allowed for the mining of datasets whose contents were not collected for a public health purpose. Data about credit card transactions is meant to justify credit card bills to credit card holders. CCTV data is normally for the protection of property against intrusion or crime. ATM data is collected to record withdrawals of funds by card users, assumed to be holders of relevant bank accounts. The fact that CCTV images and other transaction data are proxies for someone's location does not normally justify people trying to track other people's movements by those means: normally, adults have a right to move around as and when they like and to do so unobserved. The second kind of departure from norms of privacy occurred when the Korean authorities communicated more information than was necessary, including intimate information, about a Covid contact to mobile phone numbers associated with particular neighbourhoods through which an infected person passed (Zastrow 2020).

Granting that the use of intimate information was wrong, even in a pandemic, what are we to say about the repurposing for Covid track and trace of mobile phone location data, ATM and credit card transaction data, and CCTV images? The fact that quick repurposing breaks normal data protection norms is not by itself a decisive objection to what the South Koreans did, since lives and serious illness were at stake, and since numbers of lives threatened by the virus rise more steeply the longer it takes to trace spreaders of the virus and their contacts. Data protection norms are typically not broken for the sake of saving lives, and if there is no alternative, or no alternative to invading privacy in the time available, breaking a data protection norm is a considerably lesser evil than avoidably failing to prevent a death. Let us concede that even in a pandemic emergency there is no need to identify a carrier by more than the route he or she followed as he or she circulated in densely populated localities. Let us concede, too, that there is no need to exchange that location data with people who were not in the carrier's vicinity at the time. These concessions are compatible, in an emergency, with the permissibility, indeed the moral necessity, of quickly collecting and analysing a lot of relevant location data, correlating it with CCTV and ATM transaction data, and for communicating health warnings to local mobile phone numbers the authorities do not normally have legitimate access to.

It is worth pausing to consider more carefully the relative values of privacy, continued life, and continued life free of the sort of like-threatening respiratory symptoms of the worst Covid cases.

In general, privacy matters because it facilitates autonomy in circumstances in which exercises of autonomy by one person pose no risk to others. That is, in normal times, privacy helps one to lead a life determined by one's clear-headed, life-organizing, and harmless choices. (For a detailed account of the value of privacy, see Guelke and Sorell 2016.) Familiar privacy conventions block the observational and informational access of others to one's body, one's home and one's deepest opinions unless access has specifically been *granted* by the person concerned. The basic idea is that one needs a space not occupied or experienced by others in order to plan one's life freely and lead certain important parts of it satisfyingly. The freedom of individuals not to be observed, and to keep facts about themselves from becoming common knowledge, reduces the scope for manipulation or unwanted influence by others, including the state.

But the personal privacy that facilitates leading a life according to one's choices is necessarily the personal privacy of a *living person* with the capacity to choose, and the capacity to choose is dependent on one's medical condition. To put it more simply, autonomous living presupposes decision-making capacity connected to a certain level of biological functioning that medical treatment is normatively expected to maintain: pandemic emergency threatens that minimum for many in a large population. Or, in other words, autonomy depends on privacy once the medical conditions for survival and being an agent with capacity have been met. Privacy is a *less* basic good than capacity provided by normal biological functioning, and the more basic a good is, the more priority is given to each person securing it in a pandemic emergency. In this sense, the protection of life takes precedence over privacy protection when they conflict.

Facts about contagious disease in general and Covid in particular directly involve two private zones par excellence: the body and the home: the body, because Covid affects the respiratory system, and because the virus is found in noses and throats; the home, because Covid transmission involves the exhalation and inhalation of droplets by people passing close to one another in space, including, enclosed, shared domestic spaces. When homes are densely inhabited by a range of generations of the same extended family, the risk of infection and even death can be highly elevated.

Infection control in a pandemic requires the quick transmission to public health bodies of information about symptoms such as continuous coughing, fever, and the loss of one's senses of taste and smell. Normally, that is, outside emergencies, it is *not* obligatory to disclose this sort of information to the authorities. In developed countries symptom-reporting is supposed to trigger prompt testing for the virus, with positive results leading to obligatory, sometimes difficult and unpleasant, self-isolation, as well as the communication to human contact tracers of all the places and people one has recently visited. All of these obligations are privacy-violating, but are imposed for the sake of maximizing the chances of saving life and the prevention of the worst of Covid illness for the largest number. If the privacy violations are unavoidable in the time available, then they seem genuinely justifiable in the sense that inflicting the lesser of two harms when there is no other option available is justifiable.

## Test, Track, and Trace in the UK

I now turn to Covid response in the UK (The Week 2021). The main measure used by the government against the virus was a national lockdown introduced at the end of March 2020, after a short-lived and largely ineffective effort at containment. In February and early March, the UK lacked widely available large-scale testing even for workers in the healthcare sector. It had an ineffective and seriously understaffed human track and trace capacity, and its stocks of Personal Protective Equipment (PPE) for doctors and nurses in hospitals with Intensive Care Units was inadequate. It had no developed plans for assisting care homes containing what turned out to be the people most likely to die from Covid: older adults and men over 70 in particular. What is more, it transferred patients from hospitals to care homes without testing them for Covid. In these circumstances, action short of a lockdown might have produced an infection rate and a hospitalization rate that could have overwhelmed the health service in two ways: by exceeding its intensive care bed capacity, and by endangering ill-protected medical staff at the highest risk of infection and hospital-ization themselves, reducing the available medically skilled labour force in the UK (for a fuller and more forgiving account of the way UK Covid policy was developed at pace in 2020 and its relation to evidence, see Cairney 2021).

The UK Covid app was introduced as one of the elements of a test, track, and trace system with the potential to prevent further national lockdowns. What is more, it was expressly designed to leave the app user in control of data about his identity and his contacts. Downloading the app was to be voluntary, though it was also described by members of the UK government as a matter of 'civic duty' in the pandemic (The question of whether app use should be obligatory is raised in Parker et al. 2020). It was supposed to avoid requiring uniquely identifying information from the user, but transactions with the National Health Service (NHS) through the app in the event of contracting symptoms could require disclosure of part of the user's home postcode. Once downloaded onto a mobile phone, the app was supposed to exchange a big random number (its ID) with other app-bearing phones. The exchange was supposed to be occasioned by one phone with the app coming into the Bluetooth range (4–10m) of another phone with the app (see for example Ada Lovelace Institute 2020). If there was high uptake of the app, it would be much better at registering possible contacts than a single user's memory of where they had been and whom they remembered interacting with. If the adoption of the app by the public was under 60 per cent, the number of exchanges would be low, and the possibilities for contact tracing correspondingly diminished. If the uptake was high, many exchanges would potentially be recorded (Although take up of the app below 60 per cent has some effect, it is at 56 per cent and over that it has a considerable effect in conjunction with measures that reduce contact between people. See O'Neill 2020.)

The exchanged ID data was to be stored on a user's phone, and not centrally, once again as a privacy-protecting measure (NHS.UK 2020). It was not supposed to be correlated with GPS data or with phone-owner names. If the phone user started to experience symptoms that he or she thought were Covid symptoms, he or she would decide whether to share that symptom information with the NHS through the app. He or she could also decide whether to upload the stored exchanged ID data. Any exchanged ID data would be used by the NHS to inform contacts of the app user that they might have been in contact with someone who had a Covid infection. The app could ask users reporting symptoms to give further information if they wanted to, to be held centrally. The data uploaded to the app could prompt not only automated notifications to people whose apps had exchanged identifiers, but human track and trace follow-ups with the same people at the local level.

In May 2020, the app was trialled locally in the UK on the Isle of Wight. It faced a number of problems (Cellan-Jones 2020). Public uptake was below 60 per cent. The local population was older and were not very familiar with the use of apps, if they owned an appropriate mobile phone at all. There was some doubt as to whether the app worked equally well with all mobile phones, and with any Apple phones in which it operated in the 'background'. Since the decision to report symptoms centrally was left up to individual users of the app, there was no guarantee that this would be done promptly. Again, access to testing was limited, meaning that it could take a long time to answer the question whether experienced symptoms meant Covid or something else. A corresponding delay would affect the transmission of a particular user's contact history to track and trace personnel, who could begin the process of speaking to possible contacts.

Apparently for the sake of protecting privacy, then, the UK app solution afforded many opportunities for delay in the reporting of symptoms and upload-ing contacts. In the absence of a comprehensive testing programme, the UK was never likely to identify cases of infection quickly enough or trace contacts quickly enough. As a result, UK infection and death rates grew to be among the worst in the world by mid-2020. The South Korean approach not only had the important virtue of great speed which the UK approach lacked; its use of data mining also promoted privacy in some ways that the overall UK system would not. Though the South Koreans' use of high-tech tracing disclosed some embarrassing locations that carriers of the virus went to, at least the carriers did not have to admit as much to another person. *Human* track and trace can be much more intrusive because someone who experiences symptoms and tests positive is sharing intimate information with someone else—a human being—likely to be interested in the grubby details, and for whom discretion is probably far from second nature, if they have only recently been recruited to the role.

The NHS trial in the Isle of Wight exposed a number of technical and other problems with the UK app that led to its being redesigned, partly through the adoption of the up-to-then rival Apple-Google system for Covid monitoring. Although the app was eventually introduced, the whole track, test and trace system has recently been condemned by the UK House of Commons Public Accounts Committee as hugely expensive without being effective, and now that the vaccination programme has been implemented widely, the need for it is much diminished. It is one of the ironies of the post-lockdown track and trace system in the UK that the collection of personal data by people not even associated with Public Health England or the NHS increased exponentially, partly as a by-product of opening up the service economy immediately after Covid lockdown. Customers of barbershops or pubs, where close contact in confined spaces might lead to infection, were required to hand over their mobile phone numbers to barbers and barmen, so that contact tracers would be able to contact people in the event that getting a haircut or a drink brought one into contact with someone who tested positive. At least anecdotally, misuses of data grew the more data collection was done by humans. Bar staff sometimes abused the Covid data collection system in pubs by noting the phone numbers of customers they found attractive, for example (Higson 2020).

Why were the designers of the UK and other Covid apps so keen to find an alternative to the centralization of data seen in South Korea? There is some evidence that Google and Apple exerted undue influence in this area (Taylor 2021). Scruples about decentralizing Covid contact data would make sense if untrustworthy institutions or individuals would otherwise have had access to it. Large profit-making companies might come into the category of the untrustworthy, or authoritarian governments. But it is not obvious that the NHS and Public Health England—the intended possible recipients for those reporting symptoms in the UK—have the same suspect status. On the contrary, recent evidence suggests that the public in the UK overwhelmingly trusts the NHS with its health data, and prefers centralized to decentralized data collection for Covid (Maple 2020). The NHS has always held a huge stock of health data, quite apart from Covid, in the form of patient histories, most of them now in digital form, and this fact seems to provoke no public controversy whatsoever.

On the other hand, developers of decentralized apps sometimes claim that public trust is permanently fragile, and that unless data is decentralized in the case of Covid, general cooperation with the government and institutions in relation to Covid may be withdrawn (See Michael Veale's evidence to the UK House of Lords Science and Technology Committee, House of Lords 2020). Again, small-scale deliberative consultations sometimes yield general concerns about data privacy without much explanation of how these are arrived at through interactions with experts invited to present the issues (Ada Lovelace Institute 2020 The Ada Lovelace consultation was based on the contributions of twenty-eight people.).

My own view is that privacy was vastly overvalued in Covid track and trace apps. In particular, too much weight was placed on privacy in the sense of apps users' control of their own data—reflected in apps giving people the chance to refuse to report symptoms or to refuse to upload their contacts, even when app users themselves had been deidentified. Privacy is not necessarily a matter of controlling one's data but of having reliable custodians of it who control access to it on one's own behalf. This is how it is with a lot of NHS patient data, whether during a pandemic or not.

Privacy in the sense of control of one's own data makes sense where malicious actors are out to steal one's data for financial gain or use it to embarrass people. But in a public health emergency—where time is short and delays put more of a population in danger of infection and serious illness—data-sharing to promote a regime of tracing and isolation is in everyone's interest, not just the interest of an oppressive government or a data-hungry business. It is true that data sharing in these circumstances breaches data privacy norms for normal times, but this is characteristic of the morality of *emergencies*. In emergencies things that are normally not permitted may be done, and sometimes are (morally) necessary to do, to prevent imminent, major harm (see Sorell 2003; see also Sorell 2013). Of course, it makes a difference what political regime prevails where an institutional response to emergency is being undertaken. South Korea is a liberal democracy; the People's Republic of China is not. Both apparently responded effectively to the outbreak of Covid; but only the South Korean government would have been strongly accountable if containment in April 2020 had not succeeded.

Let me enlarge on these last points. Since the height of the pandemic, the Chinese government has sought to suggest origins for it outside Wuhan and indeed outside China. At least one Chinese diplomat has claimed that members of the American military brought it with them to a competitive sporting event in China (Kuo 2020). Again, the Chinese government has not been entirely cooperative with a WHO investigation of the Covid outbreak (Gan 2021). Reporting of government inaction in the early stages of the pandemic was discouraged (Allen and Feng 2020), and China silenced doctors in Wuhan who sought to publicize the illness in Wuhan in the early stages of the pandemic. In South Korea, by contrast, an idiosyncratic combination of intensive testing, high-tech tracing without scruples about privacy, and citizen cooperation produced a virtuous circle of prompt reporting, mass compliance with testing and isolation measures and avoidance of high peaks of infection and hospitalization (Kim and Kim 2020).

## An Architecture of Oppression?

We are now in a position to consider Edward Snowden's claim that Covid surveillance belongs to an 'architecture of oppression' that is to be found even in liberal democratic countries. Snowden speaks in his *Vice* interview from April

2020 of governments tracking the movements of whole populations through their mobile phones (Dowd 2020). He makes clear that he means not only East Asian but also liberal democratic Western countries, including the US.

This claim is not even *prima facie* plausible where governments themselves, such as the UK government or the Swiss government, fund Covid surveillance apps that are voluntarily downloaded, highly decentralized with respect to how data is held until the user decides, if at all, to report symptoms, and that do *not* involve bulk personal datasets. The claim is more plausible in relation to South Korea, where bulk collection did take place, and where the Covid response did show that the public health agency of the government could get quick access to these datasets. Snowden also suggested that he thought data would objectionably be retained beyond the time of the pandemic, but for purposes he did not specify (although see Henschke in this volume).

Snowden's forebodings about Covid were lent weight by his revelations in 2013 of an up to then secret use by the National Security Agency in the US of an intelligence-gathering programme (Landau 2013; Inkster 2014). The system was designed for counter-terrorism. Above all, it aimed at compiling an archive of communications data so complete that the task of finding a needle in a haystack—a previously unknown terrorist communicating with his terrorist associates—would at least not be hampered by an absence of some of the hay. The data came from the communications of US citizens with foreign nationals, and, in exceptional cases, from US citizens communicating with other US citizens. The form the data took was, roughly, records of connections between different telephone numbers or email addresses or hashtags at different times. Sometimes this is called 'contact chaining' (Gellman 2020). When this data is aggregated and subjected to network analysis, patterns of intensity of connection between different telephone numbers or other identifiers–some only indirectly connected—are revealed. Collection was supposed to proceed under warrants authorized by the Foreign Intelligence Surveillance Court, but sometimes, by the NSA's own admission, the terms of the warrants were violated.

It is possible to deny that bulk collection is seriously intrusive without denying that it is morally objectionable in other ways, and this is the approach I take. I deny that bulk collection is particularly intrusive, but I do not deny that bulk collection may be error-prone, discriminatory, and carried out on a scale that is vastly disproportionate to its success in identifying terrorists in the US. For example, only sixty-four ISIL-related arrests were made in 2014–15 (Gellman 2020), an unknown proportion of which were based on bulk collection. Not all of these arrests led to charges, and they were the meagre fruit of the collection of billions of items of communication metadata.

Even if the scale of bulk collection is disproportionate to its proven results in counter-terrorism, it may seem undeniable that bulk collection is *also* intrusive, since it is geared to identifiers that are often attached to real people, and identifying the people behind email addresses or telephone numbers is intrusive, especially if conducted on a big scale and on the identifiers of people with no connection to terrorism.

These points are reasonable enough, but they suggest inferences that might be made by nosey human investigators in a case where they have met and are curious about the suspects. Machine algorithms that identify communications links between identifiers differ from the nosey investigator in at least two ways. First, they lack consciousness, human interests, and curiosity, and second, they sift through huge datasets at very high speeds to find concealed links between identifiers—especially the kind that might reasonably be expected of terrorists trying to avoid detection by the authorities. It is true that intense communication between a terrorist suspect and someone who is only connected to the suspect romantically or commercially might register in the output of a search, but unless that contact was a security official or someone connected to a likely terrorist target, it might command no more interest than the identifier of a popular pizza parlour.

Defenders of bulk collection have often tried to counter charges of gross intrusion by distinguishing, correctly it seems to me, between metadata of telephone calls and their content, and between collection and inspection of data (for both distinctions, see Donohue 2014). One reason why this latter distinction is sometimes resisted is because two different theories of privacy are used, respectively, by defenders and critics of bulk collection. According to one theory, keeping one's data private is a matter of being *in control* of that data. Call this the *control theory*. According to the other theory, data is private until its content actually comes to someone else's attention, no matter whether it is under the control of the data subject or data producer. Call this the *attention theory*. In an earlier paper (Sorell 2018), I have defended the attention theory over the control theory.

Not much hangs on that defence of the attention theory, because what is at issue in this paper is the analogy between the mechanics of the NSA programme for counter-terrorism and a supposed 'architecture of oppression' associated with Covid. One reason why the term 'oppression' seems out of its element is that Western Covid programmes have no ambitions to 'total awareness' that the NSA once had, no ambitions to limit the freedoms of anyone beyond a short period associated with symptom reporting; and no purpose of limiting freedoms except for the sake of public health. Again, there is a world of difference between the agents of Covid data collection—public health bodies—and national security services. Further, and crucially, the *basis* for contact tracing in the NSA programme and the basis for contact tracing for Covid by virtually any government are utterly distinct.

The purpose of public health surveillance is to protect a population, usually the population of a certain jurisdiction, from infectious and other kinds of disease. Public health measures are not only in place during a pandemic, or more generally, in a recognizable emergency. They can be triggered by gradually emerging damage to health from smoking, over-eating, taking too little exercise and mass consumption of opioids. Public health measures in liberal democracies are seldom coercive; and nor are they carried out in secret. On the contrary, they are subject to journalistic inspection and criticism, government, and parliamentary oversight, and non-cooperation from patients. All of these characteristics, taken together with the authority of the science that underlies the public health measures, legitimize those measures, and surveillance to establish the effects of those measures.

Surveillance for counter-terrorism, on the other hand, is often quite different. In the NSA case, it was supervised by secret courts (the FISA courts) and applications to those courts for permission to carry out surveillance were sometimes omitted. US government oversight of surveillance operations was unsatisfactory, again for reasons of secrecy (Sorell 2018). Although US citizens were not supposed to be targets of this surveillance, they could become eligible for it if they entered into communications with foreigners, including public sector employees in other countries, even countries in security alliances with the US. This creates conditions for domination in Pettit's sense. That is, NSA surveillance made it possible in principle for the US government to exercise autonomy-threatening interference with the choices and personal or professional relationships of some of its citizens in relation to friends from friendly countries abroad. NSA activity also threatened to run counter to the spirit, and perhaps the letter, of mutual defence treaties. The personal communications of friendly foreign heads of state—Angela Merkel, for example—were intercepted (Reuters 2015). In all of these respects, NSA activity was prima facie illegitimate.

In the case of the NSA programme (Greenwald and Ackerman 2013), the US government aimed at disclosing the identities of unknown terrorists by means of electronic contacts with suspects for which there was evidence of terrorist activity. As the phrase 'needle in a haystack' implies, the NSA did not think it was easy to sift terrorist identities from vast numbers of telephone records. They assumed, very questionably, that core members of networks would emerge as focal points of communication diagrams derived from data, when, in fact, those in charge of terrorist networks—Bin Laden, for example—often communicate seldom and indirectly and not by telephone or email with those they direct.

The basis for Covid surveillance is, by contrast, much more reliable, and derived from the reputable sciences of virology and epidemiology. These sciences provide knowledge of the way the virus penetrates the respiratory system, how it is spread between people, how far it is expelled through coughs and sneezes in an interior space (Morawska et al. 2020); in conjunction with some engineering disciplines, virology can determine how the virus is affected by ventilation and temperature; how long it can survive on surfaces people touch, and so on; epidemiology can model the probabilities of exponential rises in infection rates, and so on. Among other things, all of this means that there are very solid connections between proximity of people and spread, air circulation and spread, and the path in space taken by people before and after experiencing symptoms and the locations of people on or near those paths, including cohabiting family members, staff and residents of care homes, and even strangers congregating temporarily, in bars, restaurants, airliners, and ski resorts. Virology and epidemiology have no counterparts in the social science of radicalization and the understanding of the growth and leadership of terrorist organizations. When eventually vaccines effective against new strains of Covid are sufficiently distributed and used globally, the need for contact tracing and self-isolation will decline until the next pandemic is identified. There is no analogue of this data collection pause in counter-terrorism.

## Conclusion

The arrival of a new pandemic is bad enough when it is greeted by a world ill-equipped to test for a virus and to protect those who are in the front line of treatment. To make the means of containing the virus look *sinister* is not an exercise in protecting a citizenry, but in stoking the paranoia of those on both the left and libertarian right who see ill-defined conspiracies behind quarantine, vaccine, and test, track, and trace. I do not accuse everyone who supports decentralized Covid data collection of the same paranoia. But it helps to remember in bad times as well as good that well-maintained central institutions—including the state itself—are prime means of protecting whole populations from ill health, extreme poverty, and military threat. There is no need to look for an Orwellian Big Brother behind every centralized system, including every centralized system of data collection.

## References

Ada Lovelace Institute. 2020. 'Confidence in a Crisis?' https://www.adalovelaceinstitute. org/report/confidence-in-crisis-building-public-trust-contact-tracing-app/.

Allen, Kerry, and Zhaoyin Feng. 2020. 'China Covid-19: How State Media and Censorship Took on Coronavirus'. *BBC News*, 29 December 2020, sec. China. https://www.bbc.com/news/world-asia-china-55355401.

Cairney, Paul. 2021. 'The UK Government's COVID-19 Policy: Assessing Evidence-Informed Policy Analysis in Real Time'. *British Politics* 16 (1): 90–116.

Cellan-Jones, Rory. 2020. 'Coronavirus: Isle of Wight Contact-Tracing App Trial - a Mixed Verdict so Far'. *BBC News*, 18 May 2020, sec. Technology. https://www.bbc. com/news/technology-52709568.

Cha, Victor, and Dana Kim. 2020. 'A Timeline of South Korea's Response to COVID-19'. 27 March 2020. https://www.csis.org/analysis/timeline-south-koreas-response-covid-19.

Dighe, Amy, Lorenzo Cattarino, Gina Cuomo-Dannenburg, Janetta Skarp, Natsuko Imai, Sangeeta Bhatia, Katy A. M. Gaythorpe, et al. 2020. 'Response to COVID-19 in South Korea and Implications for Lifting Stringent Interventions'. *BMC Medicine* 18 (1): 321. https://doi.org/10.1186/s12916-020-01791-8.

Donohue, Laura K. 2014. 'Bulk Metadata Collection: Statutory and Constitutional Considerations'. *Harv. JL & Pub. Pol'y* 37: 757.

Dowd, Trone. 2020. 'Snowden Warns Governments Are Using Coronavirus to Build "the Architecture of Oppression"'. 9 April 2020. https://www.vice.com/en/article/bvge5q/snowden-warns-governments-are-using-coronavirus-to-build-the-architecture-of-oppression.

Gan, Nectar. 2021. '14 Countries and WHO Chief Accuse China of Withholding Data from Coronavirus Investigation'. CNN. 31 March 2021. https://www.cnn.com/2021/03/31/asia/who-report-criticism-intl-hnk/index.html.

Gellman, Barton. 2020. 'Inside the NSA's Secret Tool for Mapping Your Social Network'. *Wired*, 24 May 2020. https://www.wired.com/story/inside-the-nsas-secret-tool-for-mapping-your-social-network/.

Greenwald, Glenn, and Spencer Ackerman. 2013. 'NSA Collected US Email Records in Bulk for More than Two Years under Obama'. *The Guardian*, 27 June 2013, sec. US news. https://www.theguardian.com/world/2013/jun/27/nsa-data-mining-authorised-obama.

Guelke, John, and Tom Sorell. 2016. 'Violations of Privacy and Law: The Case of Stalking'. *Law, Ethics and Philosophy* 4.

Higson, Steve. 2020. 'Covid-19 Threatens to Set UK Data Protection Back a Generation'. CityAM. 14 August 2020. https://www.cityam.com/covid-19-track-and-trace-data-protection-risk/.

House of Lords. 2020. 'Select Committee on Science and Technology Corrected Oral Evidence: The Science of Covid-19'. 6 July 2020. https://committees.parliament.uk/oralevidence/655/html/.

Inkster, Nigel. 2014. 'The Snowden Revelations: Myths and Misapprehensions'. *Survival* 56 (1): 51–60.

Kennedy, Jonathan. 2020. 'What Can the UK Learn from South Korea's Response to COVID-19?' *CHPI* (blog). 7 April 2020. https://chpi.org.uk/blog/what-can-the-uk-learn-from-south-koreas-response-to-covid-19/.

Kim, Taekyoon, and Bo Kyung Kim. 2020. 'Enhancing Mixed Accountability for State-Society Synergy: South Korea's Responses to COVID-19 with Ambidexterity Governance'. *Inter-Asia Cultural Studies* 21 (4): 533–41.

Kuo, Lily. 2020. '"American Coronavirus": China Pushes Propaganda Casting Doubt on Virus Origin'. *The Guardian*, 13 March 2020, sec. World news. https://www.theguardian.com/world/2020/mar/12/conspiracy-theory-that-coronavirus-originated-in-us-gaining-traction-in-china.

Landau, Susan. 2013. 'Making Sense from Snowden: What's Significant in the NSA Surveillance Revelations'. *IEEE Security & Privacy* 11 (4): 54–63.

Maass, Peter. 2015. 'Inside NSA, Officials Privately Criticize "Collect It All" Surveillance'. *The Intercept* (blog). 28 May 2015. https://theintercept.com/2015/05/28/nsa-officials-privately-criticize-collect-it-all-surveillance/.

Maple, Carsten. (2020) 2020. *SpeakForYourself.* https://github.com/carstenmaple/SpeakForYourself.

Morawska, Lidia, Julian W. Tang, William Bahnfleth, Philomena M. Bluyssen, Atze Boerstra, Giorgio Buonanno, Junji Cao, Stephanie Dancer, Andres Floto, and Francesco Franchimon. 2020. 'How Can Airborne Transmission of COVID-19 Indoors Be Minimised?' *Environment International* 142: 105832.

NHS.UK. 2020. 'Your Data and Privacy – NHS COVID-19 App Support'. Nhs.Uk. 2020. https://www.covid19.nhs.uk/.

O'Neill, Patrick Howell. 2020. 'No, Coronavirus Apps Don't Need 60% Adoption to Be Effective'. MIT Technology Review. 5 June 2020. https://www.technologyreview.com/2020/06/05/1002775/covid-apps-effective-at-less-than-60-percent-download/.

Parker, Michael J., Christophe Fraser, Lucie Abeler-Dörner, and David Bonsall. 2020. 'Ethics of Instantaneous Contact Tracing Using Mobile Phone Apps in the Control of the COVID-19 Pandemic'. *Journal of Medical Ethics* 46 (7): 427–31.

Reuters. 2015. 'NSA Tapped German Chancellery for Decades, WikiLeaks Claims'. *The Guardian*, 8 July 2015, sec. US news. https://www.theguardian.com/us-news/2015/jul/08/nsa-tapped-german-chancellery-decades-wikileaks-claims-merkel.

Roth, Kenneth. 2020. 'South Korea: Events of 2020'. In *World Report 2021.* https://www.hrw.org/world-report/2021/country-chapters/south-korea.

Sorell, Tom. 2003. 'Morality and Emergency'. *Proceedings of the Aristotelian Society* 103 (1): 21–37. https://doi.org/10.1111/j.0066-7372.2003.00062.x.

Sorell, Tom. 2013. *Emergencies and Politics.* 1st edition. Cambridge University Press.

Sorell, Tom. 2018. 'Bulk Collection, Domination and Intrusion'. In *Philosophy and Public Policy*, edited by Andrew I. Cohen. Rowman & Littlefield Publishers.

Taylor, Emily. 2021. 'The Story of the U.K.'s COVID App, and Other Pandemic Failures'. 30 March 2021. https://www.worldpoliticsreview.com/articles/29530/the-story-of-the-u-k-s-track-and-trace-app-and-other-pandemic-failures.

The Week. 2021. 'The UK's Coronavirus Timeline'. The Week UK. 30 July 2021. https://www.theweek.co.uk/107044/uk-coronavirus-timeline.

WHO. 2020. 'WHO Pandemic Phase Descriptions and Main Actions by Phase'.

WHO. 2021. 'Listings of WHO's Response to COVID-19'. 29 January 2021. https://www.who.int/news/item/29-06-2020-covidtimeline.

Zastrow, Mark. 2020. 'South Korea Is Reporting Intimate Details of COVID-19 Cases: Has It Helped?' *Nature*, March. https://doi.org/10.1038/d41586-020-00740-y

# 2

# No States of Exception

## A Neo-Republican Theory of Just Emergency Powers

*Patrick Taylor Smith*

The promise and danger of an 'emergency' is that it permits us to take extraordinary action. In various guises, some have suggested that an emergency may permit us to engineer the atmosphere (Blackstock et al. 2009), rapidly de-carbonize our economy (J. A. Miller 2020),[1] suspend *habeas corpus* (Farber 2004), and bomb civilian populations (Walzer 2015). Similarly, claims of emergency are used to justify extensive state powers in response to the COVID pandemic, from mandatory vaccination to required contract tracing and surveillance to quarantine and isolation. And, at each stage, the claim is similar: these extraordinary circumstances require extraordinary actions by the government that set aside typical legal and political safeguards. The purpose of this paper is to offer an account of when these claims are justified and when they are, for lack of a better term, tyrannical.

From Walzer's 'supreme emergency' (Walzer 2015) to Agamben's 'states of exception' (Agamben 2005) to Schmittian 'decisionism' (Schmitt 2013), emergencies are understood to permit or legitimate political agents setting aside deontological constraints—including basic rights, the rule of law, and bodily integrity—in order to pursue the common good. On this view, emergencies are qualitatively different, a normative rupture, from ordinary politics where standard values, rights, and morality are in abeyance. This, of course, generates a significant political danger: emergencies are seen to be outside 'ordinary' politics, making democratic contestation and legitimation fraught and difficult (See Agamben, whose scepticism derives from the inevitability of adopting the rupture account of emergencies. Hulme 2019).

This paper rejects this conception and argues for a continuity, both in terms of our moral obligations and political institutions, between 'normal' and 'emergency'

---

[1] The number of organizations calling for a rapid and complete restructuring of global and domestic economic systems in the name of climate emergency is too numerous to list.

Patrick Taylor Smith, *No States of Exception: A Neo-Republican Theory of Just Emergency Powers* In: *The Ethics of Surveillance in Times of Emergency*. Edited by: Kevin Macnish and Adam Henschke, Oxford University Press.

politics.[2] I argue that we should understand emergencies in the context where the need for executive discretion is foreseeable and thereby subject to a fair degree of control and legitimation. On this view, emergencies are simply different contexts for the application of justice and are defined by the extent to which those values need more or less unilateral action, more or less executive discretion, in order to safeguard or further those them. This will require carefully delineated, con-strained, and regulated arenas of executive power: a constitutional, temporary, and revocable dictatorship. In what follows, I offer a neo-republican account of just emergency powers where a more unilateral executive is a response to a changing policy environment and yet where those new powers are nonetheless constrained and non-dominating. In so doing, I borrow liberally from the oft-misunderstood institution of the Roman dictator, an example of an office with powers that are both extremely wide-ranging and yet quite limited.[3] Once we see that the *need* for emergency powers is foreseeable, then we can subject those powers to various elements of procedural justice.

## A Neo-Republican Conception of Emergency

A common view of emergencies is a three part linkage between the conceptual, the ethical, and the political. Conceptually, emergencies represent a qualitative moral departure from the ordinary, generating different values or objectives for political action. We are thereby justified in setting the moral constraints of ordinary or deontological morality aside in order to pursue the common good.[4] And *as a result of this moral distinctiveness*, we need to give political actors unprecedented or unusual authority to act unilaterally in order to take those actions, leaving standard political constraints or mechanisms of accountability aside. Let us call this linkage of the conceptual, the ethical, and the political the *Rupture Account of Emergencies* (henceforth RAE). Of course, the conceptual, moral, and the political can come apart. One could accept that emergencies do represent something fundamentally different from typical contexts but deny that they happen in ways that justify specific consequentialist principles or accept that there are special consequentialist principles for emergencies but deny that we should give execu-tives greater unilateral power in response. Yet, the RAE treats these three levels as linked, with the political powers grounded in the distinctive moral principles

---

[2] This strategy is similar, though with a greater focus on normative political theory, to (Loevy 2016). Loevy shows that emergencies are a part of 'ordinary' legal proceedings and taxonomizes the legal strategies to contain it. My later analysis takes advantage of these constraints.

[3] In using this example, I owe a large debt to (Lazar 2006).

[4] While these policy conclusions are similar to those of the 'political realists' (Geuss 2008; Williams 2005), the theoretical perspective is quite different. Realists suggest that politics has a distinct normative logic that permits leaders to do things that are morally bad, theorists who advocate for the rupture account of emergencies suggest that morality *changes* during an emergency.

which are themselves grounded in turn by the distinctive nature of emergencies themselves. This paper takes the RAE as its primary target and rejects it in its entirety: emergencies are not a qualitative departure from normal politics, rather 'normal' and 'emergency' politics lie on a continuum. Second, the moral principles that apply to normal and emergency cases are the same. Finally, greater executive discretion is justified by appeal to 'ordinary' moral principles only.

However, this rejection of RAE is consistent with the occasional defence of emergency executive powers that are quite discretionary. Since the view I defend is that we should understand the level of 'emergencyness' on a continuum, there may be extreme emergencies in which the institutional expression of the relevant emergency powers will be indistinguishable between my view and the RAE but the grounding of those emergency powers will not be a set of distinctive moral principles that apply only to emergencies.[5] So, the conceptualization will be quite different: even the justification of the most extreme 'dictatorial' powers must be made within the ordinary values of democratic politics. The continuum view is predicated on the idea that that different values can express themselves in different obligations, actions, or institutions depending on the context. To use an old example, treating Milo the Wrestler and a regular person 'equally' may require that Milo receive more food as his training burns more calories (Aristotle and Barnes 2004, 1106). Or similarly, giving everyone an equal per capita emissions budget may be a way of treating some people, depending on access to renewables and energy efficiency, unequally (Caney 2012).

If we are going to object to emergency powers, the basis of that objection will likely be that such powers constitute 'tyranny' and illegitimately constrain the freedom of those subject to them. The connotations surrounding the concept of 'dictator' similarly suggests that one reason to resist the creation of unilateral executive power free from accountability is that such power makes us unfree. One can see this concern in some states' reticence to use emergency powers to take steps to contain the novel coronavirus and corresponding protects and even violent resistance in states that have used emergency powers to declare lockdowns, curfews, travel bans, and the like.[6] Neo-republicanism, then, is a useful perspective to adopt when evaluating emergency powers.[7] Beyond representing an attractive normative ideal in its own right, neo-republican thought is useful for the analysis

---

[5] I thank an anonymous reviewer for pushing me to be clearer on the nature of the linkage between the strands of RAE.

[6] On the relationship between the Swedish constitution's guarantee of freedom of movement and its strategy of avoiding lockdowns, see (Kianzad and Minssen 2020). For just one example of significant resistance to emergency coronavirus restrictions, the Dutch Curfew riots were the worst public disturbances in decades (Van Genechten 2021). These were unusually large in scope or intensity but such resistance has been common.

[7] My view will try to be ecumenical and agnostic between the neo (Pettit 1997) and the Kantian (Stilz 2009; Ripstein 2009) variations of republicanism, as well as the related dispute between freedom as non-domination and freedom as independence. Nothing rides on these distinctions for what I say in the following.

of emergency powers in part because these emergency powers appear utterly antithetical to the neo-republican perspective. If we can provide an attractive conception of emergency powers in a normative context that is dramatically opposed to them, then that gives us some confidence that the powers and their constraints are well justified. There are several reasons why neo-republicans would be particularly sceptical of emergency powers. First, the core value of neo-republicanism is freedom; societies are just insofar as they protect and further the freedom of their citizens. Justice, legitimacy, and other political values are reducible to freedom and so the justification of coercion must be that it sustains the freedom of the coerced. Simply in virtue of this sharp focus on a single value, emergency powers cannot be justified on the need to trade freedom for some other value; the common good is defined entirely in the individual freedom of citizens.

Yet, freedom, on this view, is not merely the *absence* of interference and this is the second reason why emergency powers are difficult to justify on neo-republican grounds. A person is free, on this account, when they are not subject to the *arbitrary*, superior power of another, or domination. Two elements of this defin-ition are especially relevant here. First, one is made unfree when one under the power of another *even if* that power is not exercised in a detrimental fashion. We can imagine scenarios—the nice slaveowner, the kindly paterfamilias, the benevo-lent despot—where the unaccountable power is exercised rarely. This can be because either it is not in the powerful person's interest to exercise their power or because the subject is able to negotiate their lack of interference. For example, imagine a slave that does their labour in an exemplary fashion or manages to avoid notice and thereby is not especially bothered by their master. It is entirely up to the master whether this dynamic continues: the non-interference proceeds entirely at the whim of the master. The non-interference is not within the control of the slave and their freedom is not modally robust: the master can simply choose, without accountability, to change the equilibrium and interfere with the slave. The key element here is that the potential for interference is based upon the *arbitrary* power of another. And arbitrary, in this case, means free of accountability, contestation and control. So, a life without interference and yet characterized by the looming threat of arbitrary interference is not free and a life characterized by lawful and non-arbitrary interference designed to prevent domination is not unfree even if they are interfered with (Pettit 2011).

Thus, neo-republicanism has a complicated relationship to political power (P. T. Smith 2020). First, since political agents can wield superior power over ordinary citizens, there is a constant threat that the state will dominate if that power is exercised arbitrarily. Let's call this *public domination*. The state, then, is a potential danger in need of restraint. And what's more, a state can engage in public domination over a person *merely* by having an unchecked power regardless of whether it is used against that, or any, person. This would imply a minimalist or even anarchist conception of the state as eliminating or preventing the accumulation of superior power is one way to prevent domination. But the state, according to neo-republicanism, is morally necessary as a means to prevent *private domination*, or the domination of one citizen by another. Private individuals can find themselves with superior power over others in a variety of means—economic power, physical strength, social position—that are interconnected with political authority. What's more, without a public entity that represents the interests and will of everyone, factions, classes, and subgroups can easily come to dominate others. Or, more specifically, a smaller group can come together to dominate single individuals no matter how powerful. Neo-republicanism thus demands a public agent—the *res publica*—to have a monopoly on the legitimate use of force and extensive powers to rework the economy and enforce various norms in order to protect people from private domination.

Neo-republicanism squares the circle of both fearing and needing the state by showing that the superior power of the state can be made *non-arbitrary* by granting citizens the ability to control and direct it through a variety of legal and social mechanisms: constitutional provision of basic rights, free and fair elections, checks and balances, an independent civil society and judiciary, and the rule of law. Thus, various democratic institutions ensure that the state is non-dominating and that non-arbitrary power is then directed towards ensuring that citizens do not dominate each other through the regular and fair application of the law as well, depending on the republican theorist, economic redistribution and the support of civil society organizations. The neo-republican theory of the just state is that it represents the uniquely correct balance of concerns about private and public domination. Anarchic or minimalist states will be unable to protect people from private domination while authoritarian and non-democratic states will publicly dominate. Global governance institutions, on this view, are secondary sites of justice that exist to serve the fundamental normative interest of creating sovereign, constitutional orders that appropriately balance the need to protect citizens from public and private domination (P. T. Smith 2021; Laborde and Ronzoni 2016). Such a state will have a complicated relationship to emergency powers. On the one hand, the mere possession of power that is unaccountable to the people in the relevant ways will be enough to generate domination and the fact that such power will serve some consequentialist benefit is normatively irrelevant. On the other hand, the neo-republican state can possess powers—to enforce the law, to punish, to provide social security and other entitlements—that are not reducible to individuals even in aggregate. Collective political power, on this view, is not always a threat to freedom but rather necessary for it.

A neo-republican account of emergency is one that will explain why the political authorities and institutions should allow a greater degree of discretion in some contexts rather than others and do so using values that are legible to that specific conception of justice. To that end, I submit that a neo-republican emergency occurs due to a combination of two factors: a comparatively rapid shift in the balance of threats of public and private domination and institutional stickiness. We can imagine that current institutional equilibria are based upon various expectations about the political, social, and economic environment. Large-scale and rapid changes in that environment—such as the development of a new technology, rapid political realignment, economic depression, or the advent of a deadly virus—can change the extent to which we should be worried about public or private domination. For example, some political developments may generate a risk that the state will become more authoritarian and this may require placing greater powers with other social groups—unions, civil society groups etc.—as a countermeasure. Similarly, invasion, civil war, pandemic, famine, or other rapid shifts in the policy environment can make it so that the *relative* risk of public domination recedes while the risk of private domination rises. Therefore, the balance of reasons supports granting greater unilateral executive authority to the state to protect people from that risk. As such, in order to overcome or bypass institutional inertia—both well justified and not—in times where the threat environment shifts rapidly, the political leader needs to be able to wield power with greater discretion to ensure rapid institutional responses to changing conditions.[8]

It is important to emphasize that the shift in risk needs to relatively rapid and the precise *nature* of the risk needs to be difficult to foresee. The reason is that what makes the granting of *emergency powers* necessary is that institutions are 'sticky' and driven by complex causal processes amongst stakeholders (Wiens 2012). That is, institutions cannot be equally good at everything even within their own policy area. For example, policymakers in the United States armed forces are worried that the two-decade focus on counter-insurgency undermines their ability to fight a high intensity conflict with a peer competitor. Institutions lose personnel and forget how to do certain things well in the process of new priorities. Relearning old skills or learning new ones often means losing other capacities or doing them worse. Furthermore, stakeholders within these institutions may resist the rapid changing of their mission for self-interested or norm-governed reasons. And institutions often move slowly because they are designed to do things according to procedures and rules that have been designed with certain scenarios in mind that may be inappropriate for a rapidly changing landscape. Of course,

---

[8] An anonymous reviewer has suggested that this is another way of accepting the 'conceptual' claim of RAE since I am arguing that there is something distinctive about emergencies that we are responding to normatively, albeit with our 'normal' theories. In one sense, this is hard to deny as any account of 'just emergencies' must suggest that there is some feature that makes 'emergencies' a category worth theorizing upon. Yet, there are two important differences. First, the concept is defined in an ameliorative (Haslanger 2012) fashion—given our values, it is pragmatically useful to think about emergencies in this way—as opposed to a more descriptive analysis that suggests that emergencies are 'found' out in the world. Second, my analysis places 'emergencyness' on a continuum of contingent practical features—a polity where institutions were perfectly frictionless would have no emergencies—as opposed to a sharply delineated 'state' that one finds oneself in or not or at the extreme, in Schmittian terms, is a conceptual, logical necessity. I thank an anonymous reviewer for pushing me to clarify this.

organizations can be designed such that they learn and adapt but the process is not instantaneous and there are costs to developing that capability (For an example of how different institutional cultures enable learning, see Nagl 2005). We should not assume that institutions are instantaneously and infinitely malleable.

Both conditions are required for an emergency. If the there is no shift in the balance of threats of public and private domination, then there is no normative basis to justify the provision of greater discretionary powers to the executive; it would simply be increasing the risk or even creating public domination for no reason. On the other hand, if the relevant institutions can handle the risk without large scale rapid changes, then there is no need for greater executive discretion to deal with the threat. If the threat is sufficiently slow-moving, then institutions can develop the relevant competencies without needing to take the risk of greater unilateral authority. If the institutions can effectively respond to the threat with existing or easily gained capabilities, then likewise there is no underlying basis for greater executive authority. But it is important to see that this is a *continuum* concept. Some threats or changes in the policy environment might be represent *comparatively* greater changes in the public/private balance or, conversely require the comparatively rapid development of novel capabilities, then we should consider relatively greater executive discretion. Yet, it is never the case the foundational moral principles or considerations are set aside or that we understand ourselves to be in some radically new normative context. Rather, the same values are expressed in different ways in different contexts. So, the RAE view is false.

## The Roman Dictatorship

Of course, this does leave open the question of how this will manifest institutionally. Can we retain notions of constitutional governance and the rule of law while allowing for this kind of emergency discretion? Machiavelli, for example, argued that the occasional need for emergency powers was foreseeable even if the specific threats causing the relevant emergencies was not. Since the need for those powers was foreseeable, they could be subjected to checks and balances as well as a certain measure of popular control. A core historical example of republican governance where emergency powers were directly incorporated into the constitution is the, often misunderstood, magistracy of 'dictator' in the early Roman Republic (What follows is an amalgam generated from the following sources: Lazar 2006; Loevy 2016; Levinson and Balkin 2009).

During the Roman Revolution, various people—especially Sulla and Julius Caesar—used dictatorial powers in ways that moved far beyond their legal and constitutional authority as a fig leaf for what were, in effect, military juntas. In what follows, I will instead focus on examples in the early and mid-Republic (roughly 500–150 BCE) where the dictator operated more or less as intended. This kind of backsliding is an obvious potential risk with dictatorial powers, and I will turn towards how we can avoid that kind of devolution in our own institutions in the final section of the paper. In this section, I wish to offer a brief discussion of the institution, its powers, and its limitations. The main idea this section should convey is that the Roman dictatorship was a foreseeable, constrained, and constitutional office. The common view, starting at least with Machiavelli, that the dictator had essentially untrammelled authority to do what they wish including having the power 'over life and death' is not, strictly speaking, true though, as we shall see, the dictator's powers were quite extensive. It is important to note that given the paucity of the sources and the fact that Roman institutions were quite malleable means that there really is no such thing as *the* office of dictator; the office evolved over time. The Roman Republic was known for its proliferation of legislative venues, veto points, and sources of legitimacy as Romans rarely eliminated features of their government as opposed to adding new components as they saw fit. As a consequence, it was hard to generate unified leadership, and this led to the development and use of the dictator to 'get things done.'

In what follows, I describe the typical life cycle of the Roman dictator, though I will mark out places where the position changed over time. The process to create a dictator was initiated by a recommendation of the Senate, a body with no formal power to issue commands but with immense informal influence, especially in matters of finance and foreign policy. A consul—the magistracy with the greatest authority under normal conditions—then appointed a dictator. Most crises that lead to dictators being selected were military, but they could be called into existence to handle civil insurrections and, in rare cases, to break legislative gridlock over important matters. That is, dictators were the pinnacle of the legal hierarchy in ancient Rome, and they were the only Roman office that lacked a colleague, or a co-member of the magistracy with equivalent powers. Dictators were granted the highest *imperium* in the constitutional orbit, with the literal ability to command the bodies of those subject to their authority. In rarer cases, they exercised legislative authority, creating new constitutional arrangements if a disagreement amongst the orders of Roman society—especially between patricians and plebeians—threatened to spill into open conflict. Their power was considered so absolute that some have suggested that only *informal* norms constrained them. This absolute authority was strengthened by the legal immunity that dictator possessed during the dictatorship. It was considered remarkable when figures such as Cincinnatus gave up their dictatorship *ahead of schedule*; it reflected upon their virtuous character and their willingness to the follow the *mos maiorum* (the way of the ancestors).

Despite the ways in which the dictatorial power appeared absolute, the office was constrained and limited in several ways. First, there was separation of powers in its creation: the Senate could only recommend the appointment of a dictator, a consul had to agree. The separation of powers also extended to financial matters; the dictator did not have intrinsic authority to raise money, typically having to rely upon the Senate. Further, when creating the dictatorship for a specific circumstance, the *boundaries* of that the dictator's authorities were carefully circumscribed both geographically and in terms of policy. In the vast majority of cases, the dictator's authority only existed outside of the city of Rome—constitutional provisions banning the entrance of soldiers under arms into the city except during triumphs remained in force—and was limited to a specific issue area. In fact, the weakening of this second limitation—when Sulla was given broad discretion to change the laws and properties of the state—marked, in Roman eyes, the movement of the office towards tyranny and it faded away into irrelevance shortly thereafter. Furthermore, the various decisions and commands of the dictator remained in force only during the period of the office, which was usually limited to six months. The dictatorship then, was hemmed in by a variety of constraints that were consistent with the purpose of the office—providing unified leadership when needed—while protecting the rights of Roman citizens. The dictatorship, over time, became increasingly constrained by Roman constitutional provisions to protect what they understood to be their fundamental liberties. For example, it is likely that the dictator's *imperium* was not initially subject to the tribunician veto (or *intercesso*) and any corporal or capital punishment of Roman citizens was initially reviewable by the Roman people (*provocatio ad populum*). Yet, it seems to be—though the textual evidence is not completely clear—that both the veto and the final appeal of punishment were eventually applied to the dictatorship.

To conclude, the dictatorship was given supreme, unilateral authority but this authority was limited by the need to gain cooperation from other parts of the constitutional order for judicial enforcement and financial support, was limited geographically, temporally, and by issue area, and was constrained by constitutional provisions designed to protect the (perceived) fundamental liberties of Roman citizens. The Roman Republic eventually fell and some of the demagogues that caused its downfall used these dictatorial powers but the structural weaknesses in the Roman constitutional order and in Roman society that caused the long, slow collapse of republican liberty ran much deeper that the dictatorship. The key point for our analysis is that the dictatorship was an institution that lasted for hundreds of years—including almost 100 dictators—where the need for unilateral authority was foreseen and included within the 'normal' operation of a constitutional order in ways that included important checks upon its functioning. In the next section, I will describe a modern conception of just emergency powers that takes draws lessons from the Roman experience.

## A Neo-Republican Account of Just Emergency Powers

It is important to see that the Roman experience with dictatorship cannot be directly transposed into contemporary emergency contexts. First, the Roman constitutional order, with its focus on multiple sources of legitimacy, collegiality, and a plethora of veto points, operated to a much greater extent on norms of consensus and convergence amongst a sharply limited and hierarchically structured political class. While there could be strong differences between factions of the political class in Rome, that class was itself quite restricted in composition. What's more, nothing like modern parties and ideological conflict apply readily to Roman republican politics. Finally, constitutional orders today are much more 'coherent' in that they possess relatively unified legislative authority and legal systems. To put it another way, in the Roman world, checks and balances required that different classes of society—or groups of magistrates—each possess equivalent law-making authority while, in the modern world, the expectation is that different political institutions should be *functionally* distinguished: executive, legislative, and judicial (Pettit 2001; Skinner 1991; Lintott 2003). On one hand, this means that unilateral executive discretion is less necessary as states can be more responsive to the policy environment, using a more coherent legal system while relying upon democratic politics as a constraint. On the other hand, once unilateral authority *has* been granted to the executive, it is less restricted and state capacities to monitor and coerce are much greater (P. T. Smith 2021). So, the question becomes, 'How can we appropriately constrain an executive in the context of increased state capacity and institutional coherence without losing the effectiveness that the emergency demands?'

In what follows, I want to suggest some principles and mechanisms for maintaining accountability over executives that are granted emergency powers. First, the decision as to whether we *are* in an emergency should not lie with, or not solely with, the agency that will take on the emergency powers. In other words, there needs to be widespread political consensus across multiple components of the constitutional order that taking on emergency powers are necessary. Depending on the political order, this mechanism could work through political parties, the legislature, or the judiciary but it is key to preventing public domination that the executive cannot unilaterally seize power and then exercise it. This means that if, for example, a single party or governing coalition—of which the executive is a member—that dominates all the relevant branches of government, then the authorization of emergency powers will require more than the assent of these branches. The reason is that it would not represent a genuinely 'external' constraint on the taking and exercising of executive power. In other words, the greater the emergency power, the broader the political consensus needed to take it up. Thus, an element of the executive branch—a public health authority for example—should not be able to declare an emergency and simultaneously take up emergency powers; there should be a distinctive—if overlapping—body that determines whether there is an emergency from the agency that will execute the emergency measures.

Relatedly, it is important that the moment the emergency powers *expire* is not entirely up to the executive (see Henschke's chapter in this volume). That is, open-ended grants of discretionary power—such as the authorization of force after 9/11—need to be constitutionally prohibited (Daskal, Siemon, and Bridgeman 2020). In security or defence contexts, it was perhaps somewhat understandable to have open ended grants of power since it was likely to be obvious to everyone when the crisis passed. However, there is wisdom in the Roman practice: it is easy to let emergency grants of power become permanent and to maintain a sense of constant crisis or bureaucratic inertia, as in the War on Terror. This is especially true of public health emergencies, where the possibility of disease flare-up or return may lead to considerable vagueness as to when the 'crisis' is over. In this way, public health emergencies are much more like terrorist threats than an explicit invasion. Given this temptation, the grant of discretionary power should have an expiration date or predetermined criteria when the powers must be re-authorized by the legislature. If we use criteria—such as infection rates—then it is important to have the legislature determine clear, public criteria for when the crisis ends and to have independent agent from the executive determine when the criteria has been met and the emergency powers expire. However, if this is not possible given various epistemic uncertainties, then a strict time expiry is necessary such that the legislature must re-certify the emergency powers. Having emergency powers expire has the effect of manipulating the choice architecture on the granting and use of emergency powers, nudging decision makers in one way rather than another (Thaler and Sunstein 2009). Rather than have the default setting be that these powers remain in effect until agents within the constitutional order rescind them, the default should be that the powers will expire and that the political order must *renew* them if they remain needed. The last formal constraint is that the emergency powers must be carefully delineated to be narrowly tailored to the relevant crisis and that the ability to gather resources—especially financial resources—is not unilaterally accessible by the executive. It seems prudent to create a legislative solution in advance that sets parameters and sources of emergency funding, but all emergency funding must be democratically authorized.

The Roman dictatorship eventually included the notion that fundamental liberties of Roman citizens needed to be protected by making the office subject to the tribunal veto and popular appeal. It is important to see that these are procedural, rather than substantive, protections. A Roman citizen could be subject to corporal or capital punishment, but such an extraordinary action required some degree of popular authorization, even for the dictator. It is easy to see why, even if the Romans had a notion of basic rights, it would be difficult to enshrine them in a dictatorial context. It would be hard to predict in advance whether any potential emergency or crises could require that we give the executive discretion to set some aside in order to protect others. When Abraham Lincoln unilaterally suspended *habeas corpus*, he said, 'Are all laws but one to go unexecuted, and the Government itself to go to pieces lest that one be violated?' Of course, the provision for the suspension of *habeas corpus* was anticipated and included in the US Constitution, though without an explicit claim that the executive could active the suspension unilaterally as Lincoln did (Farber 2004). But the broad point is that we might anticipate that *some* basic liberties as envisioned in constitutional order might be suspendable in an emergency, including freedom of movement in a pandemic with an order to shelter in place. Yet, we might think that certain basic procedural rights or substantive rights are so import- ant that they cannot be subject to emergency authority. In any case, if the balance between public and private domination is such that the executive needs the authority to suspend constitutionally protected basic rights, then that power needs to be explicitly laid out and subject to democratic author- ization while at the same time being reasonably delimited. For example, it seems plausible that certain due process rights might be suspended while putting down a rebellion or invasion but that the expiration of the emergency situation snaps all prior rights back into place and so any further incarceration must be justified through normal legal channels. These constraints may be instantiated in a variety of ways in public health emergencies, but I will point to just two examples. First, it follows from this that election cancellation is prohibited and election postponement should be avoided if at all possible (Report on Election Postponement due to Covid: IDEA 2021). If this means emergency alteration of election laws in order to permit voting by mail or other practices, then this might be permissible even if such actions might violate the rule of law or explicit statute. Certain democratic participation rights are, on this view, non-negotiable. Second, these constraints would require moderate due process rights for individuals subject to coercive quar- antine. That is, if the policy is that individuals who are suspected carriers of the disease are subject to forcible quarantine, then minimal due process rights to challenge that constraint are necessary. These may not amount to normal *habeas corpus* in full legal proceeding, but basic procedural rights to challenge detention cannot be entirely alienated.

The final, and most controversial, check on dictatorial power is retrospective legal accountability. Usually, it is a considerable injustice to punish someone for a law that was passed after the relevant action or to punish someone for engaging in actions that was within their discretion. Lon Fuller (1977), for example, made the rejection of *ex post facto* rules a constitutive feature of legal systems, and it is not hard to see why for both pragmatic and intrinsic considerations. Pragmatically, laws that apply retroactively will not be effective at guiding, regulating, or directing behaviour. Intrinsically, it seems unfair to hold people responsible for actions that were not illegal. However, the emergency scenario is quite different: prospective accountability is heavily constrained by the need for discretion but retrospective accountability is not. While holding an executive legally liable for actions within their discretion if their action is judged wrong or disproportional seems unfair, the need to balance unilateral authority with accountability requires that the accountability not be subject to the strict requirements of legal culpability. In other words, the demand for 'emergency powers' activates a demand for 'emergency accountability' to ensure that such actions are non-dominating. If the emergency is indeed truly necessary, then the executive should be willing to risk the possibility of retroactive accountability in order to use the powers needed to respond to it. This accountability *need not* mean criminal liability and incarceration but include a variety of mechanisms, including civil liability, being subject to public condemnation or criticism, or prohibition from holding high office in the future. Which set of accountability mechanisms we adopt will depend on a variety of factors and the type of accountability they demand. Below, I explore what this might mean for a decision made by public health authorities to adopt interventions that have different risk profiles for different populations.

This is the logic of a certain kind of 'dirty hands' resolution (Walzer 1973 is the seminal work, and the *Stanford Encyclopedia of Philosophy* entry 'The Problem of Dirty Hands' is an excellent summary; Coady 2018). Sometimes individuals may need to violate deontic morality to avoid a catastrophe. Initially, one might think there are two potential theoretical responses to the scenario: it is permissible or obligatory to violate the deontic side constraint or it is not. Each response seems unsatisfactory and not fully responsive to the moral considerations at play: violating the deontic prescription is seriously wrong but so letting the catastrophe occur. But a hybrid position is available. The agent is justified is violating the prescription and yet we are also required to adopt the relevant social and interpersonal responses associated with wrongdoing. Thus, we adopt a sort of third category—wrong but necessary (Henschke 2016)—that must be done and yet treated as wrong by the broader moral community. Of course, our moral concepts should not behave like this under ideal conditions, but whether the preconditions obtain for the normal operation of our moral principles is not entirely under our control. Sometimes, we need to acknowledge the limits of our agency and suggest that we must respect values in the breach. Under normal circumstances, policymakers can refer to the normal mechanisms of legitimation and accountability to claim authority or moral permission to sanction and govern even when wrong on the substantive issue, but such mechanisms are relaxed in an emergency. This generates a kind of moral risk in the context of emergencies: perhaps the exercise of one's unilateral discretion will be widely accepted or normatively above reproach, but the procedural values one can appeal to when a mistake is made are in abeyance in emergencies. Executives that wish to avail themselves of emergency powers must be prepared to take that risk. *But*, it is important to see that this follows from the logic of neo-republican freedom, this category is not some special category invented for a particular class of cases but justified by same principles that require the presumption of democratic legitimacy in the first place.

Such trade-offs are not without precedent in other contexts where typical moral prescriptions are in abeyance. A soldier following *jus in bello* constraints is permitted to do things that would be wrong under 'normal' contexts. Soldiers, when captured, are not prosecuted as criminals and are supposed to be released at the end of hostilities. In exchange, however, soldiers *can* be held as prisoners of war without usual due process and they are expected to take risks with their lives to protect civilians that would be unusual and extraordinary in peacetime (for an analysis of just war conventions a kind of fair contract amongst citizens and states, see Benbaji 2008 and Statman 2014). That is, greater powers and privileges come with corresponding responsibilities. One can make a similar kind of reciprocity argument in the context of emergency powers: if one is claiming authority to exercise power with minimal prospective accountability, then one must accept greater retrospective accountability. And like our other constraints, this will operate on a continuum. The extent of qualified immunity—whether and how the exercise of discretion is protected from retrospective legal evaluation—will be determined by the breadth of the emergency powers claimed. The greater the discretion and lack of prospective accountability, the lesser the extent of immunity from retrospective legal evaluation. This will, among other things, incentivize executive agents to ask for emergency powers that are as narrowly tailored as possible to the deal with the current crisis as that will be provide them with the greatest sphere of potential immunity from *ex post facto* consequences. To illustrate how this might work in the case of corona, consider a case similar to Sweden's.[9] Imagine that some public health authority takes emergency, discretionary authority and decides to resist democratic calls for stricter lockdowns in order to pursue a herd immunity strategy and, as a consequence, the elderly population suffers very high death rates with no real compensating benefits. The public health authority—again, immune from democratic input—made a bad call. *If* the public health authority was not using its discretionary, emergency authority, then qualified immunity for making a reasonable yet bad call seems legitimate. Yet, in our case the authority *cannot* refer to normal practice of democratic legitimation to justify that immunity, so we need another check on its practice. And one way to check those officials is to make them personally liable for the consequences of their decisions. In other words, if the officials want to use their emergency authority to gamble with the lives of senior citizens, then they should have 'skin in the game' as well.

Let's end this discussion on emergency powers by discussing how these constraints may operate together in something like an unexpected global pandemic.

---

[9] It is contestable how close this is to the actual case in Sweden. But it nonetheless is true that Sweden suffered far worse death rates than its neighbours to no economic benefit as a result of a system designed to give 'experts' discretionary authority that was immunized from democratic calls for a stronger response.

Imagine that the particular dynamics of this pandemic are unforeseen, even if it was clear that governments should have been prepared for something like it. The government needs unilateral powers to limit travel, close large scale indoor events, violate privacy restrictions to engage in contract tracing, and forcibly quarantine those suspected of infection.[10] How can such unilateral powers be made consistent with individual liberty? First, we should acknowledge that the pandemic conditions make private domination—via differential risk and vulnerability to all sorts of negative impacts—more likely and these powers should be tailored to prevent that. Second, the executive should not be able to unilaterally declare emergency powers without legislative authorization. Third, the claim to unilateral power should be constrained in duration, place, and manner. The powers should be carefully delineated and need to be renewed after some reasonable amount of time. Finally, if individuals are wrongfully constrained or businesses closed ill-advisedly, they are owed compensation and damages *even if* such actions appeared justified and are within the discretionary space of the emergency powers. That is, if you use emergency powers to harm someone's interests, then good intentions or good reasons are not a defence from civil liability or political accountability. You need to be *correct*, and this kind of retroactive accountability plays a key role in sustaining non-domination in the face of unilateral power.

## Conclusion

A neo-republican view of emergencies is attractive on both theoretical and practical grounds. Theoretically, it offers a unified normative position: the constitutional order should be structured to ensure the freedom of all. It does not say that this basic moral commitment disappears when things become difficult, and in fact offers a new way of conceptualizing emergencies themselves. Thus, there is no need to take on the likely impossible task of trying to draw the line of specially where the rupture in our morality occurred: basic political egalitarianism is non-negotiable even in a crisis. On the practical side, the neo-republican account focuses our attention on institutions and accountability, offering the insight that the main issue is how to construct a constitutional order that anticipates the need for and offers the proper incentives to constrain emergency powers. We should not simply trust the virtue of executives, but nor should we ignore legitimate claims for discretion when faced with a rapidly changing environment.

---

[10] It should be noted that many states that engaged in these more coercive measures concerning coronavirus—Vietnam, Taiwan etc.—had much lower infection and death rates to the disease than European and North American nations that refused to do so out of concerns of individual liberty.

# References

Agamben, Giorgio. 2005. *State of Exception*. Chicago: University of Chicago Press.

Aristotle, and Jonathan Barnes. 2004. *The Nicomachean Ethics*. Edited by Hugh Tredennick. Translated by J. A. K. Thomson. New Ed edition. London, Eng.; New York, N.Y: Penguin Classics.

Benbaji, Yitzhak. 2008. 'A Defense of the Traditional War Convention'. *Ethics* 118 (3): 464–95.

Blackstock, Jason, David Battisti, Ken Caldeira, Diane Eardley, J. Katz, David Keith, A. Patrinos, D. Schrag, R. Socolow, and Steven Koonin. 2009. 'Climate Engineering Responses to Climate Emergencies'. *IOP Conference Series: Earth and Environmental Science* 6 (July). https://doi.org/10.1088/1755-1307/6/45/452015.

Caney, Simon. 2012. 'Just Emissions'. *Philosophy & Public Affairs* 40 (4): 255–300.

Coady, C.A.J. 2018. 'The Problem of Dirty Hands'. In *The Stanford Encyclopedia of Philosophy*, edited by Edward N. Zalta, Fall 2018. Metaphysics Research Lab, Stanford University. https://plato.stanford.edu/archives/fall2018/entries/dirty-hands/.

Daskal, Jennifer, Rita Siemon, and Tess Bridgeman. 2020. 'An Incremental Step Towards Stopping Forever War?' Just Security. 13 July 2020. https://www.justsecurity.org/71374/an-incremental-step-toward-stopping-forever-war/.

Farber, Daniel A. 2004. *Lincoln's Constitution*. New edition. Chicago: University of Chicago Press.

Fuller, Lon L. 1977. *The Morality of Law*. Revised edition. New Haven: Yale University Press.

Henschke, Adam. 2016. 'Sliding off Torture's Halo of Prohibition: Lessons on the Morality of Torture Post 9/11'. *Asia-Pacific Journal on Human Rights and the Law* 17 (2): 227–39.

Hulme, Mike. 2019. 'Climate Emergency Politics Is Dangerous'. *Issues in Science and Technology* 36 (1): 23–25.

IDEA. 2021. 'Special Reports | International IDEA'. June 2021. https://www.idea.int/news-media/multimedia-reports/global-overview-covid-19-impact-elections.

Kianzad, Behrang, and Timo Minssen. 2020. 'Sweden's Response to COVID-19: A Tale of Trust, Recommendations, and Odorous Nudges'. Bill of Health. 12 May 2020. http://blog.petrieflom.law.harvard.edu/2020/05/12/sweden-global-responses-covid19/.

Laborde, Cécile, and Miriam Ronzoni. 2016. 'What Is a Free State? Republican Internationalism and Globalisation'. SAGE Publications Sage UK: London, England.

Lazar, Nomi Claire. 2006. 'Making Emergencies Safe for Democracy: The Roman Dictatorship and the Rule of Law in the Study of Crisis Government'. *Constellations* 13 (4): 506–21.

Levinson, Sanford, and Jack M. Balkin. 2009. 'Constitutional Dictatorship: Its Dangers and Its Design'. *Minn. L. Rev.* 94: 1789.

Lintott, Andrew. 2003. *The Constitution of the Roman Republic*. Oxford University Press.

Loevy, Karin. 2016. *Emergencies in Public Law: The Legal Politics of Containment*. New York, NY: Cambridge University Press.

Miller, Jacob A. 2020. 'Stan Cox: The Green New Deal and beyond: Ending the Climate Emergency While We Still Can'. *Agriculture and Human Values* 37 (4): 1321–22.

Nagl, John A. 2005. *Learning to Eat Soup with a Knife: Counterinsurgency Lessons from Malaya and Vietnam*. New edition. Chicago: University of Chicago Press.

Pettit, Philip. 2001. *Republicanism: A Theory of Freedom and Government*. Revised ed. edition. Oxford: Oxford University Press, U.S.A.

Pettit, Philip. 2011. 'The Instability of Freedom as Noninterference: The Case of Isaiah Berlin'. *Ethics* 121 (4): 693–716.

Schmitt, Carl. 2013. *Dictatorship: From the Origin of the Modern Concept of Sovereignty to Proletarian Class Struggle*. 1st edition. Cambridge, UK; Malden, MA: Polity.

Skinner, Q. 1991. 'Machiavelli's Discorsi and the Pre-Humanist Origins of Republican Ideas'. In *Machiavelli and Republicanism*, edited by Gisela Bock, Quentin Skinner, and Maurizio Viroli. Ideas in Context. Cambridge: Cambridge University Press. https://doi.org/10.1017/CBO9780511598463.

Smith, Patrick Taylor. 2020. 'A Neo-Republican Theory of Just State Surveillance'. *Moral Philosophy and Politics* 7 (1): 49–71.

Smith, Patrick Taylor. 2021. 'A Normative Foundation for Statism'. *Critical Review of International Social and Political Philosophy* 24 (4): 532–53.

Statman, Daniel. 2014. 'Fabre's Crusade for Justice: Why We Should Not Join'. *Law and Philosophy* 33 (3): 337–60.

Thaler, Richard H., and Cass R. Sunstein. 2009. *Nudge: Improving Decisions About Health, Wealth and Happiness*. Penguin.

Van Genechten, Sarah. 2021. '"Ergste rellen in 40 jaar" in Nederland: wie zijn de relschoppers, wat drijft hen en hoe moet het nu verder?' vrtnws.be. 26 January 2021. https://www.vrt.be/vrtnws/nl/2021/01/26/rellen-in-nederland/.

Walzer, Michael. 1973. 'Political Action: The Problem of Dirty Hands'. *Philosophy & Public Affairs*, 160–80.

Walzer, Michael. 2015. *Just and Unjust Wars: A Moral Argument with Historical Illustrations*. 5th ed. Basic Books.

Wiens, David. 2012. 'Prescribing Institutions Without Ideal Theory*'. *Journal of Political Philosophy* 20 (1): 45–70. https://doi.org/10.1111/j.1467-9760.2010.00387.x

# 3

# Combating Covid-19

## Surveillance, Autonomy, and Collective Responsibility

*Seumas Miller and Marcus Smith*

Governments around the world have rapidly responded to the Covid-19 pandemic in part by using technology available to them, including metadata and social media, and developing new applications. For example, South Korea used phone metadata tracking to inform community messaging about the virus. The government published anonymized data of the locations of individuals who have contracted Covid-19, making it available to the public via websites and messaging. Depending on the population size of the locality, the specificity of these messages may allow those individuals to be identified and therefore may infringe privacy rights (N. Kim 2020a). However, it is arguable that the collective moral responsibility to combat the pandemic overrides individual privacy rights.

The provision of more specific information to the community in response to the pandemic, can be contrasted with the initial approach of extensive lockdowns that have been implemented in Europe, the United States, and Australia, which compromise individual autonomy. However, again, arguably, the collective moral responsibility to combat the pandemic overrides individual autonomy rights.

Evidently, strategies for combating Covid-19 involve a complex set of competing, and sometimes interconnected moral considerations; so hard choices have to be made. However, the idea of a collective responsibility on the part of individuals to jointly suffer some costs, e.g., loss of privacy rights, in favour of a collective good (eliminating or containing the spread of Covid-19) lies at the heart of all such effective strategies.

This chapter discusses technology responses to the pandemic and associated ethical implications. The first section focuses on the technologies used to conduct contact tracing (CT) and limit transmission of the disease. The second section discusses privacy and autonomy rights, before outlining the concept of collective responsibility and applying a theoretical framework in relation to technologies used to combat Covid-19. Throughout the chapter, the notion of function creep and the influence of the Covid-19 pandemic on the expansion of surveillance

Seumas Miller and Marcus Smith, *Combating Covid-19: Surveillance, Autonomy, and Collective Responsibility* In: *The Ethics of Surveillance in Times of Emergency.* Edited by: Kevin Macnish and Adam Henschke, Oxford University Press. © Oxford University Press 2023. DOI: 10.1093/oso/9780192864918.003.0004 technologies in modern society is considered (see also Henschke in this volume on function creep).

## Technology Responses to the Pandemic

By November 2020, the Covid-19 pandemic had infected more than 42 million people around the world, and killed more than a million (WHO 2021a). Governments adapted existing technologies and deployed phone applications to assess risk, inform decision-making, and conduct contact tracing of those who contracted Covid-19. Some phone applications utilize phone metadata to geolocate individuals, while others communicate with surrounding phones via Bluetooth to record other persons that an individual has been in close contact with. Governments have a range of existing surveillance technologies available, including closed-circuit television cameras, facial recognition technology, thermal imaging cameras, phone location metadata access, automated numberplate recognition, and financial transaction data (Servick 2020).

Covid-19 is a significant threat to public health and national security because it threatens the lives of individual citizens. A person carrying Covid-19 may be asymptomatic but a danger to others, a threat that can be avoided if reasonable measures are taken to avoid the spread. Security threats can be used by governments to make socially effective claims regarding measures to address these threats and exceptional actions to be taken beyond what would normally be acceptable (M. C. Williams 2003). Pandemics have historically fallen within this category of threat:

> Most states, as well as key international institutions, have reacted to the construction of pandemic influenza as a threat by establishing emergency planning measures, which take responses to the disease outside the realm of 'normal politics'. (Kamradt-Scott and McInnes 2012)

Governments have applied technology in response to the security threat presented by the Covid-19 pandemic. Phone applications using Bluetooth and location metadata have been developed around the world (Kamradt-Scott and McInnes 2012). A benefit of Bluetooth technology is that by communicating with surrounding phones and taking a record of those that enter a defined proximity, it does not monitor an individual's location: only their phone's relationship to other phones, mitigating the privacy concerns associated with metadata. Bluetooth data can be encrypted and deleted after a certain timeframe if there is no proximity to a positive case. Bluetooth applications have been used widely by governments in Australia, Singapore, and across Europe, as well as elsewhere, and have been accepted by large proportions of those countries' populations (Bogle 2020). However, there have been some issues with function-ality, including efficacy between the Android and iOS operating systems, and whether a phone is locked or unlocked (Bogle 2020).

The use of metadata for Covid-19 contract tracing is more controversial, as it can track a person's location whenever they have their phone in their possession, thus having greater privacy implications.[1] In South Korea, metadata has been used, and detailed descriptions of individuals' movements have been released to the public in order to enable members of the community to assess whether they may have come into contact with a person subsequently diagnosed with Covid-19 (Kim 2020a). In Israel, it was reported that a database of citizens' metadata compiled by security agency Shin Bet (and previously unknown to the public), was being used for contact tracing purposes (Halbfinger, Kershner, and Bergman 2020).

China is both the country where Covid-19 originated and a world leader in public surveillance, making it an interesting case study for the purposes of this discussion (Qiang 2019). It is well known that China has established a social credit system that uses big data integration to establish a detailed profile of their citizens and impose sanctions if they repeatedly fail to comply with social norms. This system integrates, among other forms, facial recognition and an extensive public CCTV network, phone metadata, as well as financial and medical records. It reportedly also conducts more intensive surveillance of some regions of the country inhabited by ethnic minorities (Qiang 2019).

China has implemented a compulsory smartphone application known as *Health Code*, run on the Alipay and WeChat platforms, in response to Covid-19:

> How does Health Code work? People first fill in their personal information, including their ID number, where they live, whether they have been with people carrying the virus, and their symptoms. The app then churns out one of three colours: green means they can go anywhere, yellow and red mean seven and 14 days of quarantine, respectively. The app also surreptitiously collects—and shares with the police—people's location data.   (Wang 2020)

The 700 million users of the application are required to show the colour of their app when they enter residential areas, use public transport, or enter a shopping centre; in association with their identity being verified with facial recognition technology. A controversy in China has been that authorities have not explained how the system determines the colour of someone's code, which has caused confusion for those who have received yellow or red codes without understanding why they have received the rating. One blogger stated: 'I thought the days when

---

[1] Metadata refers to information such as the location of the devices used, the phone numbers involved in a communication, and the date and time of the communication.

humans are ruled by machines and algorithms won't happen for at least another 50 years. [But] this coronavirus epidemic has suddenly brought it on early' (Wang 2020). There are suggestions that the application will continue to be used after the pandemic for public health monitoring and health care service provision, and is an example of future online government service provision (Sheng and He 2020). This further expands the already comprehensive amount of data available to the Chinese government.

Such an approach is unlikely to be acceptable to citizens in liberal democratic countries, despite the significant security threat posed by Covid-19. In Norway, the government's Covid-19 tracing application, *Smittestopp*, which utilized both GPS metadata and Bluetooth technology, was suspended after it was criticized by the country's data protection agency as inadequately balancing security and privacy risks (France-Presse 2020). In liberal democracies at least, public health responses to Covid-19 must take seriously associated equity and justice issues (Parker et al. 2020). If they do not, this will diminish trust in governments in relation to future public policy proposals. more broadly: 'Well-founded trust requires taking seriously the ethical complexities relating to the implementation of CT apps as well as being transparent about the inevitable trade-offs that are being made' (Ranisch et al. 2020, 13).

In the context of a rapidly growing technology sector offering new capabilities, applications, and devices each year, the potential for function creep and the gradual erosion of individual rights needs to be considered. As described above, the security rationale has been used in the past, such as in the context of the threat of terrorism, to introduce a range of more expansive legislation and data collection practices. There is potential for the collection of data for public health purposes to become broad and continuing. The smartphone application developed for the Covid-19 biosecurity emergency could become an ongoing requirement to prevent future pandemics and maintain public health more generally; just as the war against terrorism became a war against serious crime, and against crime in general. In that context, metadata use has expanded from initially being used by only a few police and security agencies to being used widely by governments in many Western countries (M. Smith and Urbas 2021). Function creep is a significant issue in relation to the intersection of technology developments and public policy implementation. In order to maintain trust, liberal democratic governments must ensure that data collected for a specific purpose, particularly where it is undertaken as an extraordinary measure in response to an extraordinary circumstance, it is vital that it not used for broader purposes or ways that are not transparent (M. Smith and Urbas 2021). The potential future unchecked use of surveillance technologies in liberal democracies is illustrated by the extensive data systems established in China, and in particular their use in relation to ethnic minorities (Qiang 2019, note 11).

The following part of the chapter discusses the ethical concerns for liberal democracies associated with Covid-19 contract tracing technologies. These relate to the conflicts between biosecurity, on the one hand, and privacy and autonomy, on the other. Biosecurity, and associated public health and safety, are fundamental values in liberal democracies, as in other polities, including many authoritarian ones. However, liberal democracies are also committed to individual privacy and autonomy, democracy, and therefore, democratic accountability—fundamental rights that must continue to be valued in liberal democracies. Finally, the chapter presents a theoretical framework, describing collective responsibility in the context of contact tracing technologies used to combat Covid-19.

## Ethical Analysis

### Privacy and Autonomy

The notion of privacy has proven difficult to adequately explicate. Nevertheless, there are a number of general points that can be made (S. Miller and Blackler 2017; Kleinig et al. 2012; Macnish 2018). First, privacy is a right that people have in relation to other persons and organizations with respect to: (a) the possession of information (including smartphone metadata or other data generated by a Bluetooth application) about themselves by other persons and by organizations, e.g., data stored by a telecommunications company, technology company, or in government databases, or; (b) the observation/perceiving of themselves—including of their movements, relationships and so on—by other persons, e.g., via mapping metadata to determine geolocation history or using Bluetooth application data to determine which other people a person has been in contact with. Metadata is obviously implicated in both informational and observational concerns, while data from a Bluetooth application has less significant but still appreciable privacy concerns. Further, in most countries where they have been introduced, such as Singapore and Australia, citizens can choose whether to download the Bluetooth application, while they do not have a choice if a government agency deems it necessary to access their metadata (see also Lippert-Rasmussen and Vrist Rønn in this volume).

Second, the right to privacy is closely related to the more fundamental moral value of autonomy. Roughly speaking, the notion of privacy delimits an informational and observational 'space', i.e., the private sphere. However, the right to autonomy consists of a right to decide what to think and do and, of relevance here, the right to control the private sphere and, therefore, to decide *who to exclude and who not to exclude* from it. So the right to privacy consists of the right to exclude organizations and other individuals (the right to autonomy) both from personal information, and from observation and monitoring (the private sphere). Naturally, the right to privacy is not absolute; it can be overridden. Moreover, its precise boundaries are unclear; a person does not have a right not to be observed in a public space but, arguably, has a right not to have their movements tracked via their smartphone, albeit this right can be overridden under certain circumstances. For instance, this right might be overridden if they have been directed to self-isolate in a hotel if they have recently returned from overseas—and then only for the purpose of identifying other members of the public who may have been exposed to the virus. What of persons who are carrying the Covid-19 virus and are at a risk of passing it on to other members of the community? Presumably, given the significant public health risk posed by these carriers, it is morally acceptable to utilize available data to identify these persons. If so, then it seems morally acceptable to utilize metadata to identify who these individuals may have had contact with, to isolate them and provide treatment as early as possible to reduce the chance that they will become ill and possibly die, and to reduce the number of people to whom they will pass the disease.

Thus far, we have described privacy and autonomy, considered as the rights of a *single* individual. However, it is important to consider the implications of the infringement, indeed violation, of the privacy and autonomy rights of the whole citizenry by the state (and/or other powerful institutional actors, such as corporations). Such violations on a large scale can lead to a power imbalance between the state and the citizenry and, thereby, undermine liberal democracy itself. The surveillance system imposed on the Uighurs in China, incorporating a full range of technologies including metadata, facial recognition DNA, etc. (Qiang 2019, note 11), graphically illustrates the risks attached to large-scale violations of privacy and related autonomy rights if governments use them in a discriminatory manner.

Accordingly, while it is morally acceptable to collect smartphone metadata for necessary circumscribed purposes, such as locating a missing person or in exceptional emergency situations such as the Covid-19 pandemic, it is not acceptable to collect them to establish vast surveillance states such as China, and exploit them to discriminate on a racial/political basis. However, metadata is, and arguably ought to be, available for *wider* law enforcement purposes, e.g., to assist in tracking the movements of persons suspected of serious crimes. The issue that now arises is the determination of the point on the spectrum at which privacy and security considerations are appropriately balanced. Moreover, there is the potential problem of a slippery slope and, as mentioned above, function creep.

## Collective Responsibility

As we have seen, the provision of more specific information to the community in response to the pandemic as South Korea has done, can be contrasted with the initial approach of extensive lockdowns that have been implemented in Europe, the United States, and Australia, and, of course, measures such as quarantine and enforced lockdowns compromise individual autonomy. However, arguably, the *collective moral responsibility* (Bazargan-Forward and Tollefsen 2020) to combat the pandemic overrides individual autonomy rights, (albeit restrictions on autonomy, such as lockdowns, also have deleterious economic effects).

Evidently, strategies for combating Covid-19 involve a complex set of often competing, and sometimes interconnected moral considerations (e.g., some privacy rights, such as control over personal data, are, as we saw above, themselves aspects of autonomy); so hard choices have to be made. However, the idea of a collective responsibility on the part of individuals to jointly suffer some costs, e.g., loss of privacy rights, in favour of a collective good (eliminating or containing the spread of Covid-19) lies at the heart of all such effective strategies. Accordingly, we need an analysis of the appropriate notion of collective responsibility.

One of the central senses of collective responsibility is responsibility arising from joint actions (and joint omissions). Roughly speaking, a joint action can be understood thus: two or more individual persons perform a joint action if each of them intentionally performs his or her individual action but does so with the (true) belief that in so doing each will do their part and they will jointly realize an end which each of them has and which each has interdependently with the others, i.e., a collective end (S. Miller 1992; 2001). On this view of collective responsibility as joint responsibility, collective responsibility is ascribed to individuals (S. Miller 2006); moreover, if the joint action in question is morally significant, e.g., by virtue of the collective end being a collective good or a collective harm, then the individuals are collectively *morally* responsible for it. Each member of the group is individually responsible for his or her own contributory action, and (at least in the case of most small-scale joint action) each is also individually (fully or partially) responsible for the aimed at outcome, i.e., the realized collective end, of the joint action. However, each is individually responsible for the realized collective end, *jointly with the others*; hence the conception is relational in character. As already mentioned, if the collective end of the joint action is a collective good or a collective harm, then these individual persons are collectively morally responsible for this good or harm.

Here we need to make a number of important points. Firstly, this account of collective responsibility as joint responsibility pertains not only to joint actions but also to joint *omissions*, e.g., cases in which members of a group decide not to jointly act to avoid a harm to themselves or others. Secondly, it is possible that while each participant in a morally significant joint action makes a causal contribution to the aimed at outcome of the joint action, none of these contributing actions considered on its own is either necessary or sufficient for this outcome; this is especially so in the case of large-scale joint actions involving large number of participants. Thirdly, large-scale, morally significant joint actions and omissions, such as fighting the Covid-19 pandemic, introduce a range of issues which are often not present in small-scale, morally significant joint actions and omissions. For one thing, large-scale cases often involve hierarchical organizations and hence the potential for those in subordinate positions having diminished moral responsibility and, conversely, those in leadership roles having increased moral responsibility. For another thing, the extent of the contribution to the outcome of a joint action or omission can vary greatly from one participant to another, e.g., one person might contribute by staying at home while another is a front-line health worker. Indeed, some of those who make a causal contribution to a joint action—and especially to large-scale joint actions—might, nevertheless, not be genuine participants in that joint action because in performing their contributory action they were not aiming at the outcome constitutive of the joint action; they did not have its collective end as their end.

Evidently, at least in those nation states affected, there is a collective moral responsibility to comply with reasonable measures to combat the Covid-19 pandemic and, in particular, to make use of necessary public health surveillance technologies such as phone applications to do so. The use of one or more of these applications involves, at least potentially, a cost to each individual in terms of his or her loss of privacy since, for instance, his or her movements are or might be being tracked. Moreover, there is the additional potential cost if this location data is misused by the government, or by corporations, such as Google, which governments may be in part relying upon in their efforts at pandemic surveillance. However, there is a collective good to which the use of one or more of these applications can make a significant contribution, namely, the preservation of the lives of those who would otherwise have died as a result of the pandemic (and also, indirectly, the preservation of the livelihoods of those whose jobs and businesses would otherwise have been lost as a result of the severe economic shutdown should the pandemic become widespread and ongoing).

Naturally, those who would have lost their lives had they been infected, (e.g., many elderly persons with underlying health conditions), receive a benefit, namely, their lives, that those who would have survived had they been infected (e.g., many youths with no underlying health conditions) do not receive (since they will preserve their lives, whether infected or not). However, it is by no means certain who would survive being infected and who would not, e.g., the delta variant of Covid-19 has taken the lives of many youths with no discernible underlying health conditions. Moreover, the death of large numbers of the members of a community as a result of a pandemic imposes personal (and, as just mentioned, economic) costs on those who survive the pandemic. Further, and most importantly, the survival of a large number of the members of a nation state (or other community) is surely a good of such magnitude that it outweighs the privacy costs imposed on the members of the nation state in question. Consider, for instance, that at the time of writing over one million people have died in the United States from Covid-19 compared to 3000 in the 9/11 terrorist attacks. It is self-evident that the survival of a large number of the members of a community outweighs the privacy cost to each individual member, including the privacy cost to those who would survive even if infected. Moreover, it also outweighs the aggregate privacy costs of the members of the community. Here the notion of a cooperative scheme involving a collective good and collective moral responsibility (understood as joint moral responsibility) as outlined above needs to be invoked (S. Miller 2009, 70–6).

However, in respect of cooperative schemes we need to distinguish between those in which there is a benefit to all or most who participate in it and those in which this is not the case. The obligation might seem less clear in the latter case; indeed, it might seem unfair. But consider this argument (already mentioned above):

> Sometimes an agent or agents have an obligation to conform to a scheme which burdens that agent or agents, but which significantly benefits another agent or agents. But such an obligation has little to do with the fairness of a co-operative scheme. Rather it concerns the importance or moral value of the collective end realized by the co-operative scheme. Such obligations arise, especially, in cases of need—as opposed to desire for a benefit—and the greater the need, the greater the disadvantage one ought to be prepared to suffer in order to help fulfil that need. The need in question may belong to a majority or a minority of the participants in the scheme.   (S. Miller 2001, 148)

Clearly, one such need is collective public health; a need threatened by Covid-19.

There is a further point in relation to the greater costs that might be imposed on some members of the community than on others in relation to Covid-19. Here we need to invoke the concept of a web of interdependence (S. Miller 2009: Chapter 2). In any nation state there is a complex structure of direct and indirect interdependence including across time. For instance, there is direct interdependence between employers and employees, police officers and citizens, food producers and food consumers, and so on; and there is indirect interdependence between health workers and their patients, given, firstly, patients rely on health workers but, secondly, health workers rely on their patients who may be their employers, food producers and/or police officers. Moreover, the interdependence exists across time and, indeed, across generations in so far as the older generation is now dependent on the younger and the younger was dependent on the older, and so on.

Of course, this web of interdependence is not such that meeting the needs of a single person is a necessary or sufficient condition for the meeting of the needs of any other single person, let alone of all or most other persons in a given nation state (or larger community). Rather there is a complex web of partial interdependence between individuals, between subsets, and between individuals and subsets.

This de facto web of interdependence undermines the proposition that those who are not vulnerable to Covid-19 *only* have moral obligations to those who are vulnerable by virtue of the needs of the latter, although these needs do in fact also generate obligations (as we saw above). For those who are not themselves vulnerable to Covid-19 also have needs, even if not for health protection from Covid-19. Some of these needs of those not vulnerable to Covid-19 are past needs, e.g., their past need for childcare or for a school education. Their past need for childcare or a school education was met (directly or indirectly, and individually or collectively), by parents, teachers, and others, many of whom *are* vulnerable to Covid-19. Again, some of these needs of those not vulnerable to Covid-19 are present or future needs, e.g., for present or future employment in a tourist sector decimated by Covid-19, are or will be met (again, directly or indirectly, and individually or collectively) by members of the group who *are* vulnerable to Covid-19. Accordingly, the web of interdependence generates reciprocal moral obligations among members of a nation state, and these obligations obviously include obligations to preserve the lives of their fellow members.

Naturally, there is a limit to these obligations in cases where those called upon to assist the need are required to incur significant, potentially disproportionate costs (see Macnish and Thomson in this volume for more on proportionality). The raises complex moral questions that we cannot pursue further here beyond making the point that in the case of health workers confronting Covid-19 there are stringent moral obligations on the part of members of governments in particular, as well as on citizens to ensure that the risks to these health workers are minimized. In the case of members of governments, there is the obligation, indeed collective responsibility, to provide adequate protective personal equipment (PPE) to health workers, and to design and implement public health policies and guidelines for citizens to ensure that hospitals and like facilities are not overwhelmed by Covid-19 cases, and perhaps to prioritize vaccination of healthcare workers against Covid-19. Clearly, to take one salient example, the relevant members of the former Trump administration in the US, notably former President Trump himself, failed to discharge their moral obligations in this regard. In the case of the citizens, there is the obligation, indeed collective responsibility, to comply with these public health guidelines.

To return to the collective responsibility of ordinary citizens in relation to public health surveillance technologies like phone applications, other things being equal, and assuming that the phone application(s) in question are effective (for this, see Macnish in this volume), there is a collective moral responsibility on their part to download a Bluetooth application and utilize it. Naturally, other things might not be equal. For instance, as already mentioned, the data made available to authorities might be misused. Moreover, the set of persons who are collectively morally responsible might not include all citizens (or, more broadly, all the members of the community), e.g., those who are unable to use a smartphone or who cannot afford one should perhaps be excluded (depending on whether the provision of training or smartphone is available to them at little or no cost).

Notice that, as mentioned above, this conception of collective responsibility as joint responsibility implies that each relevant person has an individual moral responsibility to download a Bluetooth application, assuming a sufficient number of the others do. Here what counts as a sufficient number of others is determined by the number required for the use of the Bluetooth to be efficacious. If hardly anyone uses the application, then I do not have an obligation to do so; since it would be pointless, because inefficacious, for me to act alone or with a tiny minority of others.

Notice also that it is not simply a matter of whether each wants to do so; rather each has a moral obligation to comply (given that others comply). However, it does not follow from this that each should be compelled to comply; it does not follow that compliance should be a matter of enforceable law. On the other hand, if the numbers who choose to comply under circumstances in which compliance is voluntary, is not sufficient to enable a Bluetooth application to be effective, then it may well be that compliance ought to be enforced by the state. For the magnitude of the harm to be avoided outweighs any given individual's autonomy in respect of using the application (as well as his or her privacy) and, indeed, the aggregate autonomy (and privacy) in respect of using the application. Moreover, the moral weight attached to the reciprocal obligations generated by the web of interdependence can also be placed on the scale in favour of enforced compliance by the state.

Further, given the questions about the functionality of Bluetooth applications and the seriousness of the threat posed by Covid-19, governments may need to resort to an option more invasive of privacy, such as analysis of metadata; and compliance with this option might need to be enforced. Perhaps—depending on the extent of the Covid-19 infection and the number of lives at risk—this should only be done in specific cases where individuals known to have the disease have placed others in the community at risk. If so, then greater, yet morally justified, moral costs (privacy and associated autonomy costs) would be imposed on members of the community. However, the government's policy in this regard would ultimately be underpinned by the collective moral responsibility of members of the community to save the lives of those threatened by the pandemic and, for that matter, to save the livelihoods of those threatened by the pandemic—since as previously noted it has become clear, contrary to many commentators, that the latter is ultimately dependent on the former. However, in the light of the example of counter-terrorist legislation enacted post-9/11, and the fact that the government already has access to a wide range of data sources about individuals, it is important that this does not lead to a normalization of the use of these phone applications introduced as an emergency measure to combat the pandemic, i.e., it is important that the infringements of privacy and autonomy in question do not continue in circumstances in which they are no longer necessary.

## Conclusion

This chapter has considered the technology responses mobilized by governments around the world to address the threat of the Covid-19 pandemic that had a significant impact on global health and economic activity in 2020. The use of smartphone metadata and Bluetooth applications have been used to assist in contact tracing and compliance with public health orders in a number of liberal democracies around the world. We have argued that there are implications for privacy and autonomy, particularly with respect to metadata (or GPS tracking) that monitor the location and movement of people, and to a lesser extent, Bluetooth applications, noting questions regarding the efficacy of the latter.

A conception of collective responsibility and of a collective good—consisting of massive harm avoidance—have been outlined that implies that there exists an individual moral responsibility to, for instance, download a Bluetooth application to reduce the threat of Covid-19 in the community. It does not follow from this that compliance should be legally required or enforced. However, if voluntary compliance is not sufficient for the application to be effective, there is an argument for enforced compliance due to the significance of the Covid-19 threat for society and the reciprocal obligations generated by the web of interdependence. With regard to more invasive measures, such as the use of metadata in ways normally limited to the investigation of serious crimes, perhaps this should be restricted to specific cases where individuals known to have the disease would likely place others in the community at direct risk of contracting the disease. However, if metadata is accessed for this purpose, it is important that this does not lead to the normalization of this approach for public health or broader purposes.

## References

Bazargan-Forward, Saba, and Deborah Tollefsen, eds. 2020. *The Routledge Handbook of Collective Responsibility*. 1st edition. Routledge.

Bogle, Ariel. 2020. 'Will COVIDSafe Keep Your Data Secure? Here's What the Experts Say'. *ABC News*, 27 April 2020. https://www.abc.net.au/news/science/2020-04-27/covidsafe-contact-tracing-app-coronavirus-privacy-security/12186044.

France-Presse, Agence. 2020. 'Norway Suspends Virus-Tracing App Due to Privacy Concerns'. *The Guardian*, 15 June 2020, sec. World news. https://www.theguardian.com/world/2020/jun/15/norway-suspends-virus-tracing-app-due-to-privacy-concerns.

Halbfinger, David M., Isabel Kershner, and Ronen Bergman. 2020. 'To Track Coronavirus, Israel Moves to Tap Secret Trove of Cellphone Data'. *The New York Times*, 16 March 2020, sec. World. https://www.nytimes.com/2020/03/16/world/middleeast/israel-coronavirus-cellphone-tracking.html.

Kamradt-Scott, Adam, and Colin McInnes. 2012. 'The Securitisation of Pandemic Influenza: Framing, Security and Public Policy'. *Global Public Health* 7 (sup2): S95–110.

Kim, Nemo. 2020. '"More Scary than Coronavirus": South Korea's Health Alerts Expose Private Lives'. *The Guardian*, 6 March 2020, sec. World news. https://www.theguardian.com/world/2020/mar/06/more-scary-than-coronavirus-south-koreas-health-alerts-expose-private-lives.

Kleinig, John, Peter Mameli, Seumas Miller, Douglas Salane, and Adina Schwartz. 2012. *Security and Privacy: Global Standards for Ethical Identity Management in Contemporary Liberal Democratic States*. ANU E Press.

Macnish, Kevin. 2018. *The Ethics of Surveillance: An Introduction*. 1 edition. London: New York: Routledge.

Miller, Seumas. 1992. 'Joint Action'. *Philosophical Papers* 21 (3): 275–97.

Miller, Seumas. 2001. *Social Action: A Teleological Account*. Cambridge, UK; New York: Cambridge University Press.

Miller, Seumas. 2006. 'Collective Moral Responsibility: An Individualist Account'. *Midwest Studies in Philosophy* 30: 176–93.

Miller, Seumas. 2009. *The Moral Foundations of Social Institutions: A Philosophical Study*. 1st edition. Cambridge University Press.

Miller, Seumas, and John Blackler. 2017. *Ethical Issues in Policing*. 1st edition. Routledge.

Parker, Michael J., Christophe Fraser, Lucie Abeler-Dörner, and David Bonsall. 2020. 'Ethics of Instantaneous Contact Tracing Using Mobile Phone Apps in the Control of the COVID-19 Pandemic'. *Journal of Medical Ethics* 46 (7): 427–31.

Qiang, Xiao. 2019. 'The Road to Digital Unfreedom: President Xi's Surveillance State'. *Journal of Democracy* 30 (1): 53–67.

Ranisch, Robert, Niels Nijsingh, Angela Ballantyne, Alena Buyx, Orsolya Friedrich, Tereza Hendl, Samia Hurst, Georg Marckmann, Christian Munthe, and Verina Wild. 2020. *Ethics of Digital Contact Tracing Apps for the Covid-19 Pandemic Response*. https://doi.org/10.13140/RG.2.2.23149.00485.

Servick, Kelly. 2020. 'COVID-19 Contact Tracing Apps Are Coming to a Phone near You. How Will We Know Whether They Work? | Science | AAAS'. 21 May 2020. https://www.science.org/content/article/countries-around-world-are-rolling-out-contact-tracing-apps-contain-coronavirus-how.

Sheng, Chuyi, and Zijia He. 2020. 'Is China's "Health Code" Here to Stay?' 18 July 2020. https://thediplomat.com/2020/07/is-chinas-health-code-here-to-stay/.

Smith, Marcus, and Gregor Urbas. 2021. *Technology Law: Australian and International Perspectives*. Cambridge New York Melbourne New Delhi SingaporeCambridge University Press: Cambridge University Press.

Wang, Maya. 2020. 'China: Fighting COVID-19 With Automated Tyranny'. 1 April 2020. https://thediplomat.com/2020/03/china-fighting-covid-19-with-automated-tyranny/.

WHO. 2021. 'Coronavirus Disease (COVID-19) Situation Reports'. 2021. https://www.who.int/emergencies/diseases/novel-coronavirus-2019/situation-reports.

Williams, Michael C. 2003. 'Words, Images, Enemies: Securitization and International Politics'. *International Studies Quarterly* 47 (4): 511–31.

# 4

# Big Data as Tracking Technology and Problems of the Group and Its Members

*Haleh Asgarinia*

## Use of Big Data Analytics to Target Persons or Groups

Digital data help data scientists and epidemiologists track and predict outbreaks of disease. Mobile phone GPS data, social media data, or other forms of information updates as epidemics progress are used by epidemiologists to recognize disease spread among specific groups of people. Given the gravity of the risk that certain groups are exposed to, restriction of movement or surveillance could be imposed on them, as we have seen in recent years. In order to control outbreaks of disease, quarantine decisions are taken based on tracking the transmission of the disease on the group level (Taylor 2016). For example, new data sources have been employed in high-stakes scenarios to track a range of life-threatening diseases, including cholera in the wake of the 2010 Haiti earthquake (Bengtsson et al. 2011), malaria transmission via network analysis (Tatem et al. 2009), and Covid-19 (this volume).

In the case of the 2010 cholera epidemics, anonymous cell phone data were used to track and predict cholera epidemics in Haiti after the 12 January 2010 earthquake. Researchers used call records to investigate population movements after cholera struck coastal towns and surrounding areas, demonstrating that many who left these areas moved to cities. This knowledge was crucial because people leaving cholera-affected areas carried the disease with them (Bengtsson et al. 2011). Mobile phone records have also provided a valuable data source for characterizing malaria transmission, enabling policymakers to modify and implement strategies for further preventing transmission (Liu et al. 2012). Using data from mobile phone networks to track population movements has therefore helped improve responses to disasters and disease outbreaks.

More recently, in response to the Covid-19 crisis, big data analytics helped public officials in making decisions about how to reopen society safely and how much activity to allow. To accomplish this, epidemiological models that capture the effects of changes in mobility on virus spread have been developed by

Haleh Asgarinia, *Big Data as Tracking Technology and Problems of the Group and Its Members* In: *The Ethics of Surveillance in Times of Emergency*. Edited by: Kevin Macnish and Adam Henschke, Oxford University Press.
© Oxford University Press 2023. DOI: 10.1093/oso/9780192864918.003.0005

reflecting on patterns of human interaction at non-residential locations of interest, such as shops, restaurants, and places of worship. The results of such findings could be used to infer which activities should be continued and which should be avoided. According to the model, infections in venues such as restaurants, gyms, and religious establishments play a disproportionately large role in driving up infection rates, restricting the reopening of such establishments, and making them a key target for control (Chang et al. 2021). As a result, big data analytics as tracking technologies can help authorities control and manage the Covid-19 pandemic and bring a premature end to epidemics.

Policymakers and authorities use information derived from big data analytics to target groups or persons. When an entity is the target of information, this means that observers, policymakers, or authorities have information that they relate to an entity in the world (Henschke 2017). The observer uses the information to target the person who is infected and the person who is at risk of infection because they have been in contact with the infected person. Moreover, the observer can target groups as potential carriers of a disease, rather than addressing persons as patients.

Though promising, pandemic surveillance brings a series of challenges for those targeted by the information derived from big data analytics. Targeting persons and groups risks causing harm to a person, as a member of a group, and to a group *qua* group. Three of the ethical issues raised by targeting a person with the information generated at the aggregate level are consent, social justice and fairness, and privacy. The negative consequences of data processing at group level are the risks of group discrimination or stigmatization. In these types of cases, the problem is not that this or that specific person has been harmed, but that the group as a whole is affected and thereby undermined (Sloot 2017). These ethical issues and harms will be discussed in the following sections.

The EU General Data Protection Regulation (GDPR) is considered a key to the successful development of technologies to tackle the Covid-19 pandemic (Mikkelsen, Soller, and Strandell-Jansson 2020; Newlands et al. 2020). The consent of a person to the processing of their health data is discussed in Articles 6 and 9. Articles 21 and 22 address concerns about discrimination. To protect a person's privacy, Article 4 identifies which types of information should be kept private. I will show that none of these principles can protect a person from the harms that arise when they are the target of pandemic surveillance. These suggest that a specific regulatory framework be developed, focusing on safeguarding information attributed to a person because they are a member of a particular group.

The cluster-type (or statistical) groupings designed by big data analytics are sources of information for making policy decisions without focusing on individual identifiability. Regarding this, obligations or regulations developed to protect individuals from the misuse of their data are not helpful at the level of the group, as groups created by algorithms or models expose those groups to potential harms without identifying individuals. Furthermore, current rules or regulations cannot protect groups against potential harms, partly because they focus on individual data protection concerns, and partly because many of the uses of big data that involve algorithmic groupings are so beneficial in furthering scientific research and improving public health. These suggest that while there are rules and obligations at the level of the individual, we must reach a stage in the development of data analytics where groups are protected against discrimination. The group should be granted privacy rights in order to limit the potential harms that can result from invasive and discriminatory data processing (Mantelero 2016). I will here investigate the feasibility of assigning group rights to the group clustered by big data analytics to mitigate harm to that group.

In the first part, I will look at the ethical issues raised by aggregate-level conclusions generated from big data that target people as members of groups, and groups *qua* groups. The second part will offer recommendations for how to improve current safeguards for persons as members of specific groups and for groups as a whole.

## Key Ethical Issues

In this section, I will first look at ethical issues raised by aggregate-level conclusions generated by or discovered from big data while targeting a person as a member of a group. Three of the ethical issues, consent, social justice and fairness, and privacy, will be discussed in this section. Second, I will look at ethical issues raised by the targeting of a group *qua* group. Group discrimination or stigmatization will be discussed in this section. I acknowledge that there are other ethical issues not listed here, and so this list is not intended to be exhaustive. However, it covers the major issues that arise in the literature.

## Ethical Concerns Raised by the Targeting of a Person as a Member of a Group

This section will deal with ethical issues that arise due to a person being targeted as a member of a group. To approach this, I will first provide a brief overview of the various types of groups created by data technologies. The distinction between different groups will enable a clearer explanation of the ethical issues. Data technologies are used to discover new patterns and relations in data. Those patterns and relations may concern numerous entities leading to profiles being formed, which in this context would be profiles of people. A profile which is a property or collection of properties of a particular group of people is known as a group profile. Group profiles are divided into two types concerning the distributivity of properties forming group profiles. First, if a property is valid for each individual member of a group, this is called distributivity or a distributive property. Second, when a property is valid for the group and for individuals as members of that group, though not for those individuals as such, this is called non-distributivity or a non-distributive property (Vedder 2000).

Distributive generalizations and profiles attribute properties to a person, or a group of people, in such a way that these properties are actually and unconditionally manifested by all members of that group. For example, having a bad health condition may be distributed among all members of a group (those who have that condition). Non-distributive generalizations and profiles, on the other hand, are framed in terms of probabilities, averages, and medians, or significant deviations from other groups. They are based on comparisons of group members with one another and/or comparisons of one group with other groups. As a result, non-distributive generalizations and profiles differ significantly from distributive generalizations and profiles. Non-distributive generalizations and profiles apply to people as members of the reference group, but these individuals do not have to display these properties in reality (Vedder 1999). For example, in epidemic research, a property may be assigned to a patient because the person belongs to a reference group, such as having a specific disease, which is non-distributive profile information, even when the patient does not get sick from the disease. In such a circumstance, the person being judged and treated is being judged and treated on the basis of belonging to the 'wrong' category of persons.

In a distributive group profile, each individual member of the group is examined, the property discovered is assigned to each member, and the group inherits the property. For example, each patient in a group is diagnosed with a certain disease based on the presence of a certain symptom, and the property is then assigned to the entire group. We can conclude that the group inherits a distributive profile shared between all members of the group. However, in a non-distributive profile, the pattern or property discovered in a group is only distributed among parts of the group. In such cases, though, the property is ascribed to each member of a group because they are the members of the group (Vedder 2000), and not because they necessarily have that property. As a result, while the probabilistic property is ascribed to the group, attribution of that property to each and every individual member is invalid because that property may or may not ascribe to a particular person in the group. For example, when a group profile states that 90 per cent of the patients in the group have a particular symptom, no one can tell on those data alone, which patients actually do have the symptom. The link connecting the non-distributive profile to the individual to whom the group profiles may apply is opaque. Hence, this type of group profiling represents a group and reveals attributes that may (or may not) be applicable to the individuals in the group, and is only applicable to the group as such (de

Andrade 2011). Thus, assigning a non-distributive group profile to a group does not imply assigning that property to each of the group's members, implying that a group and its members do not share the same property.

I can now turn to the ethical issues that arise when a person is targeted using information derived from big data analytics.

## Consent

Consent has been a point of debate and concern since its position of dominance in the post–Second World War Nuremberg Code, a set of ethical principles for human experimentation to ensure that harms to humanity like those in Nazi 'medical' experiments would never occur again (Annas and Grodin 1995; Macnish 2019). The purpose and justification of consent provisions are to provide reasonable assurance that a patient or research subject has not been deceived or coerced (O'Neill 2003). Hence, when research is aimed at impacting the conditions of its subjects, it is necessary to pay attention to research subjects' consent and awareness.

The function of consent in the big data era should be to help reduce harms associated with targeting members of a specific group. An example of potential harm perceived on group membership and not on individuals is tracking migrants fleeing a capital city in order to target cholera prevention measures (Bengtsson et al. 2011) through restriction of their travel. In this case, the question arises of how to manage big data sources in terms of consent and awareness among research subjects—as members of a specific group. To gain a better understanding of the issue, consider how group profiles are designed once more. Big data analytics are used to design group profiles to help control disease outbreaks, which are often based on fluid and contingent factors such as postal code, health status, and being in a public place at a specific time. In such cases, groups are not stable but fluid, and they are not unique or sparse but rather omnipresent and widespread. Group profiles can be designed in a fraction of a second and changed by changing the purpose and needs of grouping individuals in a specific way, so who is in and who is out of a group profile can change frequently (Floridi 2017; Sloot 2017). Thus, the issue is how to seek and obtain consent when members of a group may be unaware that they are part of a group and are included in a group because they share characteristics such as being in the same place at the same time.

In the context of big data analytics, there are two main limits to obtaining consent from those who are surveilled and grouped in a specific way. First, due to the unforeseen inferences drawn from data analytics, the possible risks and benefits might not be anticipated or anticipable at the time of initial data collection. Second, the problem stems from an inability to provide individuals with the option to choose which types of groups they want to be a part of and then make group decisions based on that. While novel approaches to consent are being developed (e.g., dynamic consent, open consent, e-consent (Budin-Ljøsne et al. 2017; Kaye et al. 2015)), there is still a lack of giving individuals the choice to decide whether to be a member of a specific group simply because they share characteristics with other members of an algorithm-designed group.

### Social Justice and Fairness

Group profiles, in this context, are designed and used only for pandemic research purposes, with guarantees that access to them is restricted to some researchers who do not share the information with others. However, things change when these guarantees are not present. The information in the profiles may then be made available to others, becoming part of the body of public knowledge in society, or the information may be used for entirely different purposes. For example, the information generated from people's health data could be used for other purposes and by third parties: for job selection procedures, insurance, loans, determining who can and cannot get back to work, or determining who can and cannot access public spaces like subways, malls, and markets (Morley et al. 2020; Sharon 2020; Vedder 2000). If this type of mission creep (Mariner 2007) occurs, then values of social justice and fairness are at stake.

Firstly, when the allocation of goods and amenities in society is based on health criteria, social justice is at issue. Generalizations and profiles can be used to help public and private entities formulate policies, or they can be absorbed into public knowledge. When the information contained in the generalizations or profiles is sensitive in nature, the situation becomes more complex because it might render members of the group vulnerable to prejudice or it may be used to make decisions regarding the allocation of scarce welfare resources. Information about people who have a high risk of developing certain diseases, especially those which may indicate a likely lifestyle, for example, can lead to stigmatization and prejudice. This information might be used to provide or restrict access to services such as insurance, loans, or jobs for members of a specific group. As a result, social justice challenges arise from some of the policy reactions to the information discovered from group profiles (Vedder 2000).

Secondly, fairness is at stake because an individual may be judged or treated based on merits or characteristics that he or she did not acquire voluntarily, such as a poor health condition. However, because the feature is one of the group and not necessarily of the individual, a person as such may not exhibit or even experience those characteristics at all. This occurs when non-distributive generalizations and profiles are used instead of distributive generalizations and profiles.

### Privacy

Data technologies are used to find patterns or relationships in a dataset through maximizing dissimilarities between groups and optimizing similarity within a group (Aouad, Le-Khac, and Kechadi 2007). As mentioned above, the patterns or relationships uncovered could apply to various entities, resulting in the formation of individual or group profiles. Group profiles may be used to infer characteristics to individuals (Henschke 2017). For example, the aggregation of data may result in the knowledge that those with low oxygen saturation may be more likely to be infected with Covid-19. Thus, algorithms design a group with low oxygen saturation, which is labelled as having a high risk of infection. Consider the case where a person's data were collected, stored, and processed, and the information 'low oxygen saturation' is attributed to him or her. This information might help clinicians make early decisions regarding the arrangement and organization of medical resources and early interventions to improve the health outcomes of this patient (Benito-León et al. 2021).

However, inferring group characteristics to individuals threatens the privacy of the individual as a member of a group. Inferred information tells us something about individual members of those groups in a very qualified way (Vedder 2000), assuming that the information is produced in a sound and reliable way. When an individual member intends to keep that information private, or when the information inferred is contrary to an individual member's preference, the privacy of members, rather than individual privacy, is threatened. The reason for this is that issues of individual privacy arise when the information generated is uniquely about a specific individual, meaning that the link between that individual and the information generated is strong. However, there are privacy issues when the link between the information generated and that individual is weak, especially in a non-distributive group profile, meaning that the information produced could have been formed from another source. In such cases, privacy claims are derived from group claims following the aggregation of the data (Henschke 2017). As a result, given the lack of direct connection to the individual source, inferring group characteristics to individuals in situations where a person is a data source threatens the privacy of members, implying that a more in-depth examination of how the privacy of groups' members is considered in the context of data protection is required.

## Ethical Concerns Raised by Targeting a Group *Qua* Group

In this section, I will look at group discrimination or stigmatization when a group is targeted. Consider an epidemic that appears to target certain minorities disproportionately, resulting in additional restrictions being imposed on those minority groups, regardless of whether members of the group have the disease. In what follows, group discrimination or stigmatization will be discussed.

Contact tracing apps, GPS ankle monitors and other wearables, cell phone location data collection, genomic testing, and targeted quarantines, among other bio-surveillance technologies being used to respond to the Covid-19 pandemic, have the potential to exacerbate discrimination against racial minorities and immigrants. As a result of the Covid-19 pandemic, racial disparities in health outcomes have increased, while communities of colour, immigrants, and other marginalized groups have been blamed for spreading the disease. Disturbing disparities in Covid-19 surveillance of racial minorities have emerged, for example, in the United States. In New York City, Black or Latinx people made up 92 per cent of those arrested for violating Covid-19 protocols, such as social-distancing requirements. Black people were targeted by government authorities at four and a half times the rate of White people for such violations (Sundquist 2021). As a result of 'inappropriate surveillance' (Macnish 2012), certain population groups, namely immigrants and certain non-White racial groups, are discriminated against and blamed for disease outbreaks, which may represent a biased evaluation and become a source of social discrimination.

Making inferences and drawing conclusions about groups based on an extensive collection of information threatens the group's privacy because revealing this information increases the risk of potential harm to the group itself. Hence, the surveillance technologies used in the fight against Covid-19 have an impact on the privacy of some groups, such as marginalized communities. That is, even if all members of a marginalized group are individually protected from unwanted intrusion and targeting, the group as a whole is not protected against disproportionate surveillance, implying that individual privacy can be effectively protected while the group as a whole is not adequately protected.

Consider a situation in which each individual knowingly shared his or her data and agreed to the type of processing to be performed at the time. Assume that the lawfully obtained and lawfully processed set of personal data enabled an analyst to draw sophisticated inferences—say, on the likelihood of disease outbreaks among populations—predicting the behaviour of a group of individual data subjects as a group. Such inferences would be based not on analysing past individual behaviour to predict future individual behaviour, but rather on comparing and contrasting the behaviours of all members of a group defined by one or more shared characteristic (Kammourieh et al. 2017). Disclosing information discovered about a group therefore increases the risk of harm to that group's privacy because it increases the risk of discrimination against the group.

## Current Measures to Address the Identified Issues

In this section, I will look at the current guiding regulation regarding data protection, the General Data Protection Regulations (GDPR), to explore the suitability of existing legal frameworks to address and mitigate the identified issues. I demonstrate that further work is required to address the identified issues and that specific rules or regulations need to be developed that differ from those already existing regulations in the field of data protection.

## Protecting Persons against Harms

Article 9 provides the legal ground for special categories of personal data in the context of epidemics. Processing of special categories of personal data, such as health data 'for reasons of public interest in the area of public health, such as protecting against serious cross-border threats to health' is allowed. These special categories of personal data are processed for reasons of public interest without the consent of the data subject. This Article is unable to address the identified consent issues and instead introduces a new issue in the form of the privacy–health trade-off.

Profiling and discrimination concerns are reflected in GDPR, especially in Article 21. This Article introduces the right of data subjects to object to personal data processing, including profiling, at any time. If the purpose of data processing is direct marketing, the data subject will have an absolute right to object (Wachter 2018). However, the scope of the Article is limited to individual profiles that analyse or predict specific aspects of natural persons without taking into account harms that arise when a person is considered as a part of a whole group, particularly non-distributive group profiles in which the analysis or prediction is performed by comparing and contrasting the behaviour of all members of a group, rather than predicting behaviour of a specific person based on his or her available data.

Article 4(1) determines which types of information are protected by GDPR. Personal data allowing for identification of a natural person, including online identifiers or factors specific to the physical, physiological, genetic, mental, economic, cultural, or social identity of that natural person, are protected. Nevertheless, as soon as the data have ceased to be personal data in the strict sense, it is not clear how the principle should be applied. For example, the right of controlling data does not apply to information derived from personal data (Vedder 2000). As a result, in the age of big data and information inferred, the interest in informational privacy no longer provides sufficient protection to the *individual members of a group*; it focuses solely on information collection rather than analysis of *aggregation data* (Kammourieh et al. 2017).

In order to address the issues, we need to rethink and expand our current moral vocabulary and legal frameworks for dealing with information technology. Broadening the scope of information protected by the right to privacy and data protection to include information primarily attributed to a person because of their membership in a specific group is one way to address the shortcomings of current privacy conceptions in relation to big data analytics (for more information, see Vedder's definition of categorical privacy (1999)). Furthermore, Henschke (2017) and Kammourieh et al. (2017) propose the protection of metadata, the valuable information that can be inferred from datasets, rather than raw data, as a way to address privacy issues.

## Protecting Groups against Harms

According to Mantelero (2016), group privacy is the right to limit the potential harms to the group itself that can derive from invasive and discriminatory data processing.[1] At the group level, the right to privacy can be perceived as a duty of the state not to use its powers arbitrarily. A group right to privacy prevents the arbitrary use of power, such as discriminating illegitimately between different groups in society or exercising power for no reason at all (Sloot 2017). Understanding group privacy in terms of protecting groups against the possible negative consequences of generalizations and profiles cannot be reduced to individual privacy, meaning that the protection of group members cannot protect the group itself.

It could be asserted that, in some cases, the protection of individuals can protect specific groups. GDPR, for example, has the potential to provide safeguards against groups. GDPR provides enhanced protection for certain types of highly sensitive data, including 'revealing racial or ethnic origin, political opinions, religious or philosophical beliefs, trade union membership, and [ ... ] the processing of data concerning health or sex life' (Art. 9, EU Parliament 2016). While this is a protection granted to the individual, its effect is also to protect specific groups that are more vulnerable to targeting (Kammourieh et al. 2017). As a result, GDPR has the potential to limit the discovery of information about existing groups, such as racial groups.

However, GDPR is mainly focused on protecting individual identity and on safeguarding personal information. In an era of big data, where information about groups is extracted from data, or where more information is discovered about existing groups, the individual is often incidental to the analysis. Thus, the problem is not that this or that specific person has been affected, but that groups have been harmed. Since the group is exposed to the risks derived from the creation and use of inferred data, the infringement takes place at the group level while the rights and remedies are granted at the individual level (Kammourieh et al. 2017; Taylor, Floridi, and Sloot 2017; Sloot 2017). Regarding this, it is important to assign rights to a group to protect that group against discriminative harms. Granting this right to groups is different from the existing right in the field of privacy and data protection, in that this right to privacy is not reducible to the privacy of the individuals forming such groups.

There are at least two reasons why group rights to privacy cannot be reduced to individual rights to privacy. First, the training set used to develop a model and then generate an inference may not include all members of the group (e.g., patients with a specific disease), implying that, while there is no violation of the individual right (because members of the training set provided full informed

---

[1] It is assumed that the group right to privacy is limited to the right against discrimination.

consent to the collection, analysis, and inference of the data), there is a violation of the right to the broader group, i.e. (the set of all patients with the same disease) minus (the set of people of the same disease in the training set). Second, the information discovered by big data analytics may be targeted at specific groups comprising different individuals with diverse interests. Due to this, the group's interests[2] should fulfil the individual interests of diverse members at the same time: those who have no interest in limiting their information usage and those who do. Consequently, the group's interests may not correspond to the interests of each individual member, meaning that the group's interests are not the result of the aggregation of its members' individual interests. Irreducibility of the group's interests to a simple aggregation of individual interests implies that the group's right to privacy must be invoked to protect non-aggregative group interests.

The preceding discussions highlight the importance of developing group rights to privacy to address issues that revolve around the risks of discrimination and the adverse outcomes of big data analysis. In what follows, I will discuss the feasibility and problems of ascribing group rights to privacy to a clustered group.

## Group Rights to Privacy

So far, I have discussed that, in contrast to how privacy has traditionally been conceived on an individual level, the era of big data raises new questions about privacy on a group level. In such cases, access to personally identifiable information of individuals is less likely to cause harm. Harm is more likely to occur when authorities or corporations draw inferences about people on a group level. As a result, the concept of privacy must be stretched and reshaped in order to help us think about groups. Floridi (2014) was the first to bring up the concept of group privacy in relation to big data analytics insights. He argued that it is crucial to investigate whether groups have privacy rights that are not reducible to the privacy of the individuals who make up those groups.

According to Floridi's argument, a group's right to privacy is a right held by a group *qua* group rather than its member severally; it is referred to as a group right in the *strong* sense, the corporate approach to group rights. Right-holding groups are conceived as moral entities in their own right, with a being and status similar to that of an individual person. This viewpoint holds that a group has an identity and existence distinct from its members. Accordingly, *unity* and *identity* are necessary for a group to be the type of group that can bear rights (French 1984; Newman 2011; Taylor et al. 2017; Taylor & Floridi 2017). For example, French

---

[2] According to the choice (will) theory of rights, to have a right is to have a choice, so it makes sense to ascribe rights only to beings who are capable of choice (Hart 1982). Since clustered groups clearly lack the capability of choice, I limit myself to the interest (benefit) theory of rights.

(1984) contends that the Gulf Oil Corporation's rights and responsibilities in purchasing or selling property, or in being responsible for environmental pollution and cleaning it up, are not reducible to the individuals currently associated with it. Organizations of this type have identities that are not exhausted by the identities of the people who work in them; one person leaving and another joining does not form a new organization. As a result, a group's unity or identity distinguishes it as the type of group that might have rights.

However, proponents of group rights in the *moderate* sense, the collective approach to group rights, such as Raz (1988), argue that groups are not conceived as having independent standing, but rather as having rights shared in and held jointly by the group's members, rather than being a mere aggregation of rights held by the group's members individually. The individuals who comprise the group have a right that none of them have as independent individuals. In this view, collective rights are ascribed to a specific collection of individuals because there are some sorts of public goods that can only be held by the collective. In respect of the public production of such goods, participants in a participatory activity possess collective rights. For example, the provision of a cultured society requires participation amongst members of the group; each individual needs others in order to produce the desired society. Accordingly, there is no individual right to a cultured society, but rather participants in a joint action possess collective rights (Miller 2001; Raz 1988).

I argue that, in the case of a group designed by algorithms or data technologies, it is implausible to regard a group's right to privacy as a group right in either the strong or moderate sense. The reason for this is that in this kind of group, the essential criteria for both strong and moderate approaches on group rights to privacy are not met. On the one hand, because of the lack of integrity or unity needed to hold a right according to strong approaches, a group's right to privacy cannot be described based on these approaches. A group's right to privacy, on the other hand, cannot be conceived based on moderate approaches because members of the relevant group cannot perform a joint action to produce any good simply because they cannot realize the condition required to constitute a joint action, which is 'believing that their action is dependent on the action of other members' (Miller 2001: 57).

Although a group's right to privacy (for a group designed by algorithms) cannot be explained theoretically using either strong or moderate approaches to group rights, we can take methodological approaches to justify why a cluster-designed group requires such a right. For this, I propose employing constructivist theories implying that the need for a moral group's right to privacy is practical. According to such theories, any reason that justifies a right as a moral right must be morally neutral (Copp 1995). Thus, the justification of a moral right must be explained by invoking non-moral values. From this perspective, I claim that a group designed by algorithms would be rationally required to have a group's moral right to privacy to meet its non-moral values, if any, associated with such a right. For example, we need to grant a right to privacy to a clustered group to protect health (or sensitive) information about that group in cases where revealing or releasing that information about the group affects the members' relationships with others in society.

## Conclusion and Recommendations to Improve Current Measures

Big data analytics have the capacity to uncover new information, find patterns, and predict behaviour, allowing for the algorithmic creation of totally new groups. In this regard, it is necessary to reconceptualize the risk of data harm to include the problem of the group and its members. For researchers, it is difficult to manage the source of big data regarding consent and awareness on the part of research subjects. A further problem is that the application of data technologies undermines the values of social justice and fairness, since an individual may be judged or treated on characteristics they did not acquire voluntarily (or at all). Finally, because data technologies are used to target people as members of specific groups rather than individuals, they are increasingly threatening group members' privacy rather than individual privacy. In addition to the issues that arise when a person as a member of a specific group is targeted by the information derived from a group profile, there are also risks to the privacy of a group *qua* group because revealing the information about a group increases the risk of discrimination against that group.

In order to protect groups as such, I agree with Floridi (2014) that clustered groups must have rights to privacy which do not reduce to the privacy of individuals forming such groups. I also agree with Mantelero (2016) that a group right to privacy is required to limit the potential harms that can result from invasive and discriminatory data processing. However, group rights to privacy cannot be theoretically ascribed to a clustered group using traditional approaches. In terms of the significance of granting such rights, I recommend taking a methodological rather than predominant standard approaches to interpret moral group rights to privacy.[3]

## References

Andrade, Norberto Nuno Gomes de. 2011. 'Data Protection, Privacy and Identity: Distinguishing Concepts and Articulating Rights'. In *Privacy and Identity Management for Life*, edited by Simone Fischer-Hübner, Penny Duquenoy, Marit

[3] Haleh Asgarinia is supported by the PhD fellowship from the 'PROTECT—Protecting Personal Data Amidst Big Data Innovation' project, funded by the European Union's Horizon 2020 research and innovation programme under the Marie Sklodowska-Curie grant agreement No. 813497.

Hansen, Ronald Leenes, and Ge Zhang, 352:90–107. IFIP Advances in Information and Communication Technology. Berlin, Heidelberg: Springer Berlin Heidelberg. https://doi.org/10.1007/978-3-642-20769-3_8.

Annas, George J., and Michael A. Grodin, eds. 1995. *The Nazi Doctors and the Nuremberg Code: Human Rights in Human Experimentation*. New York: Oxford University Press.

Aouad, Lamine M., N. Le-Khac, and M. Kechadi. 2007. 'Lightweight Clustering Technique for Distributed Data Mining Applications'. In *Industrial Conference on Data Mining*. https://doi.org/10.1007/978-3-540-73435-2_10.

Bengtsson, Linus, Xin Lu, Anna Thorson, Richard Garfieldarfier, and Johan Schreeb. 2011. 'Improved Response to Disasters and Outbreaks by Tracking Population Movements with Mobile Phone Network Data: A Post-Earthquake Geospatial Study in Haiti'. *PLoS Medicine* 8 (August): e1001083. https://doi.org/10.1371/journal.pmed.1001083.

Benito-León, Julián, Ma Dolores del Castillo, Alberto Estirado, Ritwik Ghosh, Souvik Dubey, and J. Ignacio Serrano. 2021. 'Using Unsupervised Machine Learning to Identify Age- and Sex-Independent Severity Subgroups Among Patients with Covid-19: Observational Longitudinal Study'. *Journal of Medical Internet Research* 23 (5): e25988. https://doi.org/10.2196/25988.

Budin-Ljøsne, Isabelle, Harriet J. A. Teare, Jane Kaye, Stephan Beck, Heidi Beate Bentzen, Luciana Caenazzo, Clive Collett, et al. 2017. 'Dynamic Consent: A Potential Solution to Some of the Challenges of Modern Biomedical Research'. *BMC Medical Ethics* 18 (1): 4. https://doi.org/10.1186/s12910-016-0162-9.

Chang, Serina, Emma Pierson, Pang Wei Koh, Jaline Gerardin, Beth Redbird, David Grusky, and Jure Leskovec. 2021. 'Mobility Network Models of Covid-19 Explain Inequities and Inform Reopening'. *Nature* 589 (7840): 82–7. https://doi.org/10.1038/s41586-020-2923-3.

Copp, David. 1995. *Morality, Normativity, and Society*. Oxford: Oxford University Press.

EU Parliament. 2016. *Regulation (EU) 2016/679 of the European Parliament and of the Council of 27 April 2016 on the Protection of Natural Persons with Regard to the Processing of Personal Data and on the Free Movement of Such Data, and Repealing Directive 95/46/EC (General Data Protection Regulation) (Text with EEA Relevance)*. OJ L. Vol. 119. http://data.europa.eu/eli/reg/2016/679/oj/eng.

Floridi, Luciano. 2014. 'Open Data, Data Protection, and Group Privacy'. *Philosophy & Technology* 27 (1): 1–3. https://doi.org/10.1007/s13347-014-0157-8.

Floridi, Luciano. 2017. 'Group Privacy: A Defence and an Interpretation'. In, 83–100. https://doi.org/10.1007/978-3-319-46608-8_5.

French, Peter A. 1984. *Collective and Corporate Responsibility*. New York: Columbia University Press.

Hart, H. L. A. 1982. 'Legal Rights'. In *Essays on Bentham*. Oxford: Oxford University Press. https://doi.org/10.1093/acprof:oso/9780198254683.003.0008.

Henschke, Adam. 2017. *Ethics in an Age of Surveillance: Personal Information and Virtual Identities*. Cambridge: Cambridge University Press. https://doi.org/10.1017/9781316417249.

Kammourieh, Lanah, T. Baar, J. Berens, E. Letouzé, Julia Manske, J. Palmer, David Sangokoya, and P. Vinck. 2017. 'Group Privacy in the Age of Big Data'. In. https://doi.org/10.1007/978-3-319-46608-8_3.

Kaye, Jane, Edgar A. Whitley, David Lund, Michael Morrison, Harriet Teare, and Karen Melham. 2015. 'Dynamic Consent: A Patient Interface for Twenty-First Century Research Networks'. *European Journal of Human Genetics* 23 (2): 141–6. https://doi.org/10.1038/ejhg.2014.71.

Liu, Jiming, Bo Yang, William K Cheung, and Guojing Yang. 2012. 'Malaria Transmission Modelling: A Network Perspective'. *Infectious Diseases of Poverty* 1 (November): 11. https://doi.org/10.1186/2049-9957-1-11.

Macnish, Kevin. 2012. 'Unblinking Eyes: The Ethics of Automating Surveillance'. *Ethics and Information Technology* 14 (2): 151–67. https://doi.org/10.1007/s10676-012-9291-0.

Macnish, Kevin. 2019. 'Informed Consent'. In *Data, Privacy and the Individual*, edited by Carissa Veliz. Madrid: IE University Press.

Mantelero, Alessandro. 2016. 'From Group Privacy to Collective Privacy: Towards a New Dimension of Privacy and Data Protection in the Big Data Era'. In, 139–58. https://doi.org/10.1007/978-3-319-46608-8_8.

Mariner, Wendy K. 2007. 'Mission Creep: Public Health Surveillance and Medical Privacy'. SSRN Scholarly Paper ID 1033528. Rochester, NY: Social Science Research Network. https://papers.ssrn.com/abstract=1033528.

Mikkelsen, Daniel, Henning Soller, and Malin Strandell-Jansson. 2020. 'Data Privacy in the Pandemic | McKinsey'. 2020. https://www.mckinsey.com/business-functions/risk-and-resilience/our-insights/privacy-security-and-public-health-in-a-pandemic-year. *Account*. Cambridge: Cambridge

Miller, Seumas. 2001. *Social Action: A Teleological Account*. Cambridge: Cambridge University Press. https://doi.org/10.1017/CBO9780511612954.

Morley, Jessica, Josh Cowls, Mariarosaria Taddeo, and Luciano Floridi. 2020. 'Ethical Guidelines for Covid-19 Tracing Apps'. *Nature* 582 (7810): 29–31. https://doi.org/10.1038/d41586-020-01578-0.

Newlands, Gemma, Christoph Lutz, Aurelia Tamò-Larrieux, Eduard Fosch Villaronga, Rehana Harasgama, and Gil Scheitlin. 2020. 'Innovation under Pressure: Implications for Data Privacy during the Covid-19 Pandemic'. *Big Data & Society* 7 (2): 2053951720976680. https://doi.org/10.1177/2053951720976680.

Newman, Dwight. 2011. *Community and Collective Rights: A Theoretical Framework for Rights Held by Groups*. 1st edition. Hart Publishing.

O'Neill, O. 2003. 'Some Limits of Informed Consent'. *Journal of Medical Ethics* 29 (1): 4–7. https://doi.org/10.1136/jme.29.1.4.

Raz, Joseph. 1988. *The Morality of Freedom*. Clarendon Paperbacks. Oxford: Oxford University Press. https://doi.org/10.1093/0198248075.001.0001.

Sharon, Tamar. 2020. 'Blind-Sided by Privacy? Digital Contact Tracing, the Apple/ Google API and Big Tech's Newfound Role as Global Health Policy Makers'. *Ethics and Information Technology*, July. https://doi.org/10.1007/s10676-020-09547-x.

Sloot, Bart van der. 2017. 'Do Groups Have a Right to Protect Their Group Interest in Privacy and Should They? Peeling the Onion of Rights and Interests Protected Under Article 8 ECHR'. In, 197–224. https://doi.org/10.1007/978-3-319-46608-8_11.

Sundquist, Christian Powell. 2021. 'Pandemic Surveillance Discrimination'. *SETON HALL LAW REVIEW* 51: 13.

Tatem, A., Y. Qiu, David L. Smith, O. Sabot, Abdullah S. Ali, and Bruno Moonen. 2009. 'The Use of Mobile Phone Data for the Estimation of the Travel Patterns and Imported Plasmodium Falciparum Rates among Zanzibar Residents'. *Malaria Journal*. https://doi.org/10.1186/1475-2875-8-287.

Taylor, Linnet. 2016. 'Safety in Numbers? Group Privacy and Big Data Analytics in the Developing World'. SSRN Scholarly Paper ID 2848825. Rochester, NY: Social Science Research Network. https://papers.ssrn.com/abstract=2848825.

Taylor, Linnet, and Luciano Floridi. 2017. 'Group Privacy: New Challenges of Data Technologies'. *Group Privacy*, 293.

Taylor, Linnet, Luciano Floridi, and Bart van der Sloot. 2017. 'Introduction: A New Perspective on Privacy'. In *Group Privacy: New Challenges of Data Technologies*, edited by Linnet Taylor, Luciano Floridi, and Bart van der Sloot, 10–22. Philosophical Studies Series. Cham: Springer International Publishing. https://doi. org/10.1007/978-3-319-46608-8_1.

Vedder, Anton. 2000. *Law and MedicineCurrent Legal Issues Volume 3*. Edited by Michael Freeman and Andrew Lewis. Oxford University Press. https://doi.org/ 10.1093/acprof:oso/9780198299189.001.0001.

Vedder, Anton. 1999. 'KDD: The Challenge to Individualism'. *Ethics and Information Technology* 1 (4): 275–81. https://doi.org/10.1023/A:1010016102284.

Wachter, Sandra. 2018. "Normative Challenges of Identification in the Internet of Things: Privacy, Profiling, Discrimination, and the GDPR." *Computer Law & Security Review* 34 (3): 436–49. https://doi.org/10.1016/j.clsr.2018.02.002.

# 5

# Epistemic Dimensions of Surveillance in Public Health Emergencies

## Risks of Epistemic Injustice and Dysfunctions of Trust

*Katrina Hutchison and Jane Johnson*

## Introduction

Public health emergencies—whether they be pandemics, natural or human-caused disasters—give rise to distinct knowledge needs and sometimes justify new or invasive forms of data gathering and surveillance to meet these needs. In a pandemic, these can be aimed at protecting individuals, protecting the health system or economy, reducing or controlling overall case numbers or spread, predicting and managing outbreaks, or enforcing pandemic-related legislation. In other types of emergencies—such as a bushfires, hurricanes, and terrorist attacks—different forms of information gathering might be helpful. In particular, these disasters often require information to assist with locating and identifying individuals and providing safe, effective healthcare to displaced persons in hospitals and makeshift care environments where there may not be access to the usual technology.

In this chapter we focus on the knowledge-related aspects of surveillance for public health emergencies. We argue that distinctive features of public health emergencies can give rise to epistemic injustices including testimonial injustices and dysfunctions associated with trust. If unaddressed, these threaten not only the fairness and moral acceptability of the public health response but also the epistemic goals of public health surveillance. That is, inattention to epistemic injustices in public health emergencies can undermine the ability of authorities to collect essential data needed to manage the emergency and ensure public safety.

The chapter is divided into three parts. In the first part we map some features of public health emergencies, and how these give rise to distinctive epistemic challenges. We use a case study of the Australian New South Wales State government's response to the COVID Delta outbreak to illustrate these features.

Katrina Hutchison and Jane Johnson, *Epistemic Dimensions of Surveillance in Public Health Emergencies: Risks of Epistemic Injustice and Dysfunctions of Trust* In: *The Ethics of Surveillance in Times of Emergency*. Edited by: Kevin Macnish and Adam Henschke, Oxford University Press. © Oxford University Press 2023. DOI: 10.1093/oso/9780192864918.003.0006

In section two we introduce the concepts of epistemic injustice as understood by Miranda Fricker, and testimonial smothering as described by Kristie Dotson, and outline how these can occur in the context of public health surveillance. Epistemic injustices are wrongs to an individual in their capacity as a knower, which arise due to negative identity-prejudicial stereotypes—e.g., racist, sexist, or homophobic stereotypes that interfere with judgements of credibility (Fricker 2007). We argue that in the case of contact tracing or enforcing pandemic-related legislation, the word of some individuals might be treated as highly credible, whereas the word of members of some marginalized groups may be treated as far less credible. This has implications for which geographic locations surveillance measures are implemented in, how and where surveillance measures are enforced, and the interpretation of discrepancies between surveillance data and individuals' own accounts of their movements and health. There is potential for this to unfairly discriminate against members of some oppressed groups. Moreover, it can have implications for the quality of data and thus the generation of knowledge essential to managing the public health emergency. We continue to use the case of the New South Wales Covid-19 Delta outbreak to illustrate these challenges.

In section three, we explore epistemic challenges associated with trust. Drawing on work by Annette Baier and Katherine Hawley, we argue that the epistemic injustices described in section two occur against the background of racist and classist prejudices that shape trust relationships between authorities and citizens. In particular, groups who already distrust healthcare and law enforcement authorities due to past systemic injustices may be more likely to distrust or attempt to subvert surveillance measures. Moreover, authorities may be more likely to apply extensive surveillance backed by police enforcement in areas populated with marginalized groups due to prejudices. These prejudices include credibility deficits as well as expectations that some populations will be less likely to follow public health orders, and more likely to attempt to evade or subvert surveillance measures. We argue that this produces a vicious cycle that is both unfair and threatens the ability of authorities to generate knowledge essential for managing the public health emergency for the safety of all citizens.

## Some Features of Public Health Emergencies, and Their Implications for Knowledge

In the context of public health, the World Health Organization (WHO) defines surveillance as 'systematic ongoing collection, collation and analysis of data for public health purposes and the timely dissemination of public health information for assessment and public health response as necessary' (World Health Organization 2016). Surveillance in public health contexts can take a range of forms and serve various ends. Peter Nsubuga and colleagues (2006) note that this can range from active surveillance for immediate use—as in the detection/management of newly emerging health problems, to passive collection of information used for understanding the natural history of diseases or setting research priorities (see Nsubuga et al. 2006: Table 53.1).

Here, our focus is on the forms of public health surveillance utilized in public health emergencies (although, as we will argue, the distinction between emergency and routine surveillance may be difficult to maintain). In this section we ask: what are the features of public health *emergencies* (as opposed to non-emergency contexts) that interact with the *epistemology* of public health surveillance to produce specific challenges?

Several features of public health emergencies are relevant for understanding the epistemological challenges of surveillance in these contexts and the risks of associated epistemic injustices.

1. Public health emergencies are *acute* deviations from normal for the health-care system. They share this feature with some other, non-emergency events, such as mass gatherings.
2. Public health emergencies involve *significant risks* to the health of individuals. They share this feature with other, non-emergency public health issues, including lifestyle diseases such as type 2 diabetes.
3. Public health emergencies are unplanned and unpredictable. They are not scheduled, and it is difficult to predict whether and to what extent future emergencies will share features with past emergencies.

Each of these features produces distinctive challenges for officials. The acute nature of public health emergencies means that emergency measures are likely to be temporary, needing to be implemented quickly when the emergency arises and drawn to a close at an appropriate point after the emergency situation has been brought under control. Identifying the 'end' of an emergency is not necessarily clear-cut. One challenge, noted in other chapters in this volume (see, for example, Henschke [Chapter 9 in this volume]), is whether, when and how measures put in place to respond to temporary challenges during an emergency will be unwound when the critical period has passed. In some cases, the knowledge requirements associated with the public health emergency are temporary. For example, knowledge requirements for contact tracing during a disease outbreak are only required during the outbreak.

In contrast, despite the acute nature of the emergency some knowledge-related goals served by surveillance systems during a public health emergency do not have an end point. For instance, in the aftermath of Hurricane Katrina, there was widespread discussion of the role that modern surveillance technologies and/or big data systems could play in avoiding future systemic failures during disasters.

One recommendation was wider uptake of public health records and/or mobile health records. Many people displaced by flooding sought treatment from providers who did not have access to their medical histories and health records. Moreover, some physical records were destroyed. A centralized system of electronic health records, or a system of mobile health records accessible by patients, can potentially mitigate the harms and risks of treating displaced people (Irmiter et al. 2012; Bouri and Ravi 2014). However, a system set up to mitigate against these risks would only work if it was ongoing and set up prior to, and independently of, any particular emergency.

Experiences gained during managing one event, may lead to maintaining rather than unwinding surveillance systems developed. Sarah Thackway and colleagues from the New South Wales Department of Health (Thackway et al. 2009), describe a decade of progress by public health officials in Sydney, Australia, in utilizing surveillance processes to manage public health risks associated with hosting mass gatherings. During the decade they describe, processes implemented for the Sydney 2000 Olympics and Paralympics, and 2003 Rugby World Cup are built upon rather than unwound. They describe, for instance, how systems developed during the Rugby World Cup underpinned success in identifying and mitigating outbreaks of influenza and gastroenteritis during the 2008 World Youth Day in Sydney. The paper provides an argument for maintaining and strengthening (rather than unwinding) surveillance mechanisms implemented during one acute public health event to boost preparedness for future events. The same arguments could be applied to at least some emergency surveillance mechanisms.

The serious risks associated with public health emergencies mean that it is critically important officials make the 'right' decisions. The immediate and the ongoing health and even the lives of large numbers of people can depend on public health responses. Yet the other features of public health emergencies—notably their unpredictability—mean that making the right/best decisions is challenging. Unpredictability means that whilst readiness/planning and preparation should be informed by past emergencies, there is no guarantee that this will be adequate for future demands. Moreover, the planned-for emergency might never arise, thus any preparations are at risk of being a waste of effort and resources. If there are ethical risks or harms associated with planning—for example, risks of depleting scarce resources, polluting the environment, or violating citizens' privacy—then these risks or harms may be in vain if undertaken for a prepared-for emergency that never eventuates.

From the perspective of epistemology, it is important to note that the combination of these three features (acuteness, serious risk, and unplanned/unpredictable nature of emergencies) means public health emergencies are associated with epistemic (knowledge) gaps and a rapidly shifting epistemic environment. What is known about an emerging illness, new epidemic, or unfolding natural or human-caused disaster can change rapidly. In a rapidly changing epistemic environment public health officials have to keep in mind that they are making decisions based on limited information, which may later be judged with the benefit of hindsight and much more comprehensive knowledge. It is important for officials to be honest about the limits of their knowledge and the unfolding nature of the situation, so that they can maintain public trust both at the time and when decisions are viewed in hindsight. Communication of important facts as currently understood, alongside communication about the limits of knowledge and the rapidly changing epistemic situation, must be accomplished quickly.

The New South Wales state government response to the 2021 outbreak of the Delta strain of Covid-19 in Australia provides a helpful case study for understanding some forms of surveillance and how they are used alongside other information-gathering techniques to meet various knowledge needs. The government's response to the outbreak made extensive use of multiple different surveillance technologies alongside other methods, outlined in Table 5.1.

These methods can loosely be grouped into three 'types' of information gathering for the purposes of our argument.

(1) Non-surveillance (contact tracing interviews, police checkpoints)—which provide detailed fine-grained information about individuals with the potential to fill gaps or correct errors in surveillance data.

(2) Bespoke surveillance—purpose-built systems like QR scanner-based systems to gather location data for contact tracing, digital handshake-based location systems to gather data for contact tracing (e.g., Australia's COVIDSafe App), sewage surveillance, genomic sequencing, and mandatory surveillance testing of specific populations.

(3) Appropriated/co-opted surveillance—using data collected for other reasons (google/facebook movement data), or surveillance equipment installed for other reasons (security footage, numberplate scanning) to meet emergency-related information needs.

Table 5.1 highlights a number of points: the diversity of methods used to gather information, how several methods can be used together (e.g., for contact tracing), and how these information-gathering activities deliver knowledge needed to pursue various goals.

A distinction can be made between primary public health–related knowledge needs—such as knowledge requirements for contact tracing, diagnosis and linking of cases—versus secondary knowledge needs that support the public health response. These secondary supports include the enforcement of public health orders by law enforcement officials. For simplicity, we will think of the primary knowledge needs as those delivered by health officials and healthcare workers, and we will think of secondary knowledge needs as those delivered by other authorities such as law enforcement in their pandemic-related activities. Some of the surveillance activities in Table 5.1 *could* inform both activities.

**Table 5.1** Information-Gathering Methods and their aims, NSW Covid-19 Delta Outbreak, 2021

| Aim/Goal | Method (Data Gathering Technique) |
|---|---|
| Identify areas in which there are cases | Surveillance of sewage in areas of concern to identify the presence of cases[1] |
| Identify cases and measure extent/trends of outbreak | **Bespoke mandatory surveillance testing** of individuals from some groups, e.g., essential workers from Local Government Areas (LGAs) of concern who need to leave those LGAs for work |
| Identify contacts of cases | **Contact-tracing interviews** with positive cases[2] |
| | **Digital surveillance systems such as Australian COVIDSafe App**[3] |
| | **Bespoke 'check-in' processes** which tracked which businesses/sites people were visiting via a process of checking in using a smartphone QR code scanner. |
| | **Use of existing data that records check-ins** (e.g., opal cards, passenger logs on flights) |
| | **Use of existing surveillance equipment at locations** (e.g., security camera footage) to identify the movements of infected individuals in crowded spaces[4] |
| Identify/confirm links between cases | Genomic sequencing to establish whether cases are linked |
| Understand movement patterns and measure impact of restrictions | **Use of existing movement data** captured by tech companies such as Facebook and Google to understand the impact of restrictions on movement of people[5] |
| Control movement and deter rule-breaking | Checkpoints on roads Number plate scanning |

[1] In the 1940s in the United States studies of poliomyelitis virus in sewage demonstrated the relationship between rates of infection in the community and levels of virus in wastewater (Melnick 1947). From 1988 sewage surveillance became a cornerstone of the Global Polio Eradication Initiative (Asghar et al. 2014). In NSW, the chief health officer is the one who determines sewage testing locations based on areas of concern. (Health Protection NSW 2023)

[2] Note that interviews often make use of electronic data of various kinds—for example, asking people to check their internet bank records for transactions at shops. Contact tracers could also ask you to check your text messages, social media post, and photos as prompts. (Curtis and Clun 2020; Housen 2020)

[3] For further details about the COVIDSafe app, see Degeling et al. 2021. The COVIDSafe app was one of the tools available to NSW Health during the outbreak. However, at 30 September 2021, COVIDSafe app had not uncovered any close contacts in the most recent outbreak, according to media sources. (Conifer 2021)

[4] The use of security camera footage was widely reported in the Australian media at the time, as reflected in this article from the national broadcaster: (Calderwood 2021)

[5] As for other methods, this was reported in local media: (Hanrahan 2021)

Using surveillance technologies to inform public health decision-making poses several costs and risks, including: financial cost of gathering, processing, and acting on the data; financial and other costs of safely storing data or destroying it when no longer needed; opportunity costs if inappropriate method is selected; risks of privacy/security breaches; risks associated with data linking; and risks associated with public perceptions and trust in authorities.

Given these costs and risks, there are some common-sense epistemic demands we might make regarding surveillance. For one thing, the goals of the surveillance must be important and acceptable to the community. Second, if surveillance is worth doing at all it is worth doing adequately—there is no point collecting data unless it will serve the purpose for which it is collected. This means the surveillance system and process must be designed to collect *at least* the minimum amount of data required to achieve the goal. On the other hand, because some risks (privacy, security, and data linking) may be higher with more invasive or extensive surveillance, the system should gather no more data and be no more extensive than necessary to achieve the goals. Similar principles are outlined in early articles on disease surveillance (e.g., Foege, Hogan, and Newton 1976).

Unfortunately, these common-sense demands are somewhat naïve and out-dated in the context of modern surveillance technologies, where electronic health records, insurance claims data, registry data and other forms of routine data are often co-opted and sometimes linked to serve a range of different ends. The New South Wales (NSW) management of Covid-19 Delta outbreak illustrates several ways that authorities co-opt surveillance data gathered for other purposes to fill knowledge gaps in an emergency.

Another principle is in tension with the common-sense demands. Knowledge and truth are widely regarded as intrinsically valuable (Nevo 2010). This might imply that there is normative/moral pressure to maximize the knowledge generated by surveillance data in health contexts. Murdoch and Detsky talk about a 'transition of data from refuse to riches' (2013: 1351), implying that it would be wasteful not to maximize the knowledge from collected health data. Porsdam, Savulescu, and Sahakian (2016) argue that the duty of easy rescue applies to use of data from electronic health records for research: when someone can save another person at almost no cost to themselves, they ought to do so. However, different intuitions come to the fore when a significant moral wrong has occurred in the collection of the data—e.g., data from medical experiments undertaken in Nazi concentration camps, or with the remains of Nazi victims. Some of the Nazi data was based on methodologically flawed science, or did not generate original results, but some appears to provide unique, valid results with potential applications.[6] The methods used to obtain this data are universally decried. However, there has been

---

[6] Moe (1984) uses the example of data on hypothermia, and Yee et al. (2019) focus on Pernkopf's Atlas of Anatomy, which includes anatomical illustrations from the remains of Nazi victims.

robust discussion about whether it is morally permissible to use or cite the results. On one hand is a view that using these results could 'salvage some good' (Moe 1984: 7) given that the data has already been collected and the victims are no longer suffering. In contrast, some scholars deny the moral permissibility of *ever* citing or using this data (e.g., Post 1991). Researchers have also challenged the acceptability of deriving important knowledge from other morally questionable data—for instance Rebecca Tuvel argues that if animal experimentation is morally wrong, then the use of data from past animal experiments is also wrong (Tuvel 2015). These cases show that even if knowledge has intrinsic value, the 'refuse to riches' logic of Murdoch and Detsky can be resisted: it does not follow that data must never be 'wasted'.

Our focus is emergencies. Some of the abovementioned features of emergencies—such as the acute state of significant risk, and the epistemic/knowledge gaps—can give licence for collection or use of data to fill the knowledge gap in ways that would normally be more rigorously scrutinized. For example, there were cases of reduction in oversight during the Covid-19 pandemic (Blakely et al. 2022). Despite this, we question the extent of exceptionalism about emergencies when it comes to co-opting surveillance data. Big data and eHealth data are *often* co-opted for public health purposes outside of emergencies (e.g., Tu et al. 2015; Lamarche-Vadel et al. 2014; Kupersmith et al. 2007). These uses may need to be approved by an ethics committee, but they do not typically require consent from the individuals whose data is utilized. If those individuals consented at all, it is likely to have been a one-off broad consent authorizing use of the data for a wide range of possible future purposes.

Researchers have described trends in the rise of data driven science generally as well as in health contexts. There has been some debate over whether analysing big data sets is a new way of doing science, with significant implications for the scientific method (e.g., Frické 2015; Leonelli 2014; Mazzocchi 2015; Canali 2016). In the context of public health research, there has been significant discussion of the potential benefits and risks of co-opting surveillance and eHealth data for public health purposes. For instance, Samerski argues that the distinction between public health and personal clinical healthcare is being eroded by big data. Personal electronic health records increasingly produce data utilized in public health and medical research (Samerski 2018). In an article reflecting on big data ethics and epistemology, Lipworth et al. (2017) provide a list of examples of sources and uses of such data which suggests, as Samerski argues, that the gap between routine and emergency/special purposes for data collection may be closing. One Health approaches to emerging infectious diseases recommend more integrated collection of surveillance data on human and animal diseases, as well as their links to environmental conditions such as climate change, changes in patterns of interaction of humans and animals, and encroachment of built environment (e.g., Johnson, Hansen, and Bi 2018; Johnson et al. 2019). Within this wider context, there is both an abundance of data available to be co-opted for use in public health emergences (and/or systems in place to collect it). These examples suggest that it may be increasingly difficult to distinguish exceptional uses of surveillance data that are characteristic of public health emergencies from routine practice in public health. Surveillance is used on an ongoing basis to monitor safety, disease patterns, and to ensure preparedness for mass gatherings. Moreover, co-opting of routine medical data (such as insurance claims data and electronic health records) for non-emergency public health research is becoming common. As such, the most distinctive thing about public health emergencies might be the licencing of other interventions such as public health orders and associated law enforcement mechanisms.

## Testimonial Injustice and Testimonial Smothering in Public Health Emergencies

In the previous section we outlined/mapped some features of public health emergencies and described how these pose distinctive epistemic needs and challenges. We also outlined some of the ways that surveillance is used alongside other data to meet these challenges. We noted the increased use of modern surveillance technologies in public health, as well as increased utilization of co-opted data captured for other reasons to inform routine public health activities. For this reason, emergency situations are increasingly similar to routine public health activities in terms of at least some surveillance measures. In fact, the most distinctive feature of emergencies (compared to routine contexts), from a public health surveillance perspective is the collaboration with other officials—especially law enforcement officials—to enforce public health orders in the face of unexpected and serious health risks.

In this section, we argue that the epistemic challenges associated with meeting knowledge needs in public health emergencies include risks of testimonial injustice and testimonial smothering of individuals from oppressed groups. These risks are heightened by the relationships between public health officials and law enforcement officials in emergencies. As in the previous section, we draw on examples from NSW's response to the 2021 Covid-19 Delta outbreak.

What are epistemic injustices? According to Miranda Fricker (2007), 'distinctively epistemic' injustices affect an individual in their capacity as a knower. Fricker identifies two varieties of epistemic injustice. Hermeneutical injustices occur when someone lacks the conceptual resources to describe or communicate their experiences, due to unjust social arrangements. Fricker's example of this is the challenge women faced in describing their experiences of sexual harassment before consciousness-raising during the women's movement led to the naming and conceptualization of this type of harm. Testimonial injustices occur when someone is unjustly deemed to know more or less about a subject matter than they do, based on identity prejudicial stereotypes. Specifically, they occur when uptake of someone's testimony does not match the reliability of that testimony due to negative identity-prejudicial stereotypes. These often involve individuals suffering credibility deficits when they try to share their knowledge on particular topics.

In Table 5.1, above, we summarized some of the knowledge aims and data-gathering methods involved in the NSW response to the 2021 Covid-19 Delta outbreak. Some knowledge goals listed in the table are served by more than one data-gathering technique. For example, contact tracing relies on a mix of personal interviews with positive cases, and data from surveillance methods. Where public health officials mesh different types of information together in this way, especially when combining information from personal interviews with information from various surveillance sources, there are risks of testimonial injustices.

Contact tracing processes are typically private, so it cannot be expected that there are specific examples of these sort of testimonial injustices described in the public domain. However, it is easy to construct a hypothetical example where surveillance data contradicts individuals' own accounts of their movements. Suppose a woman is shown on surveillance data from a QR Code check-in system to have visited a café in violation of lockdown restrictions while symptomatic with an illness later diagnosed as Covid-19. The woman denies that she visited the café and claims that she never violated the lockdown restrictions. She suggests that a family member who cares for her children and with whom she sometimes shares a mobile phone may have inadvertently checked in using her details rather than their own. A testimonial injustice will occur if authorities decide similar cases differently—for instance if they gave the benefit of the doubt to the testimony of an educated or wealthy white woman in this situation, but not to the testimony of a non-white migrant or someone who appears less well educated or less well off.

The tension between two different ways the contact tracing information might be used are clear in this case. Officials engaged in contact tracing have an interest in eliciting comprehensive and honest testimony from positive cases, in order to notify all close contacts. However, if positive cases are anxious that their interview responses may be used by law enforcement officials to sanction violations of public health orders, this might tend to impact on the completeness and truthfulness of testimony. This could be true despite it being illegal for contact tracers to share information with law enforcement officials—people's beliefs, expectations, and degree of trust in the authorities do not always track the facts about how the information is used (Housen 2020). A catch-22 can arise if individuals with marginalized social identities who have good reason to distrust officials are *expected* to give flawed testimony, and in turn, they modify what they say due to perceiving that they are not fully believed. In the next section, we offer a more detailed analysis of the dynamics and risks of this sort of mutual distrust.

Kristie Dotson (2011) has described a similar but different phenomenon of 'testimonial smothering', whereby a speaker from an oppressed group cuts short her testimony because she doesn't think it will receive proper uptake from the audience. She outlines three conditions:

> 1) the content of the testimony must be unsafe and risky; 2) the audience must demonstrate testimonial incompetence with respect to the content of the testimony of the speaker; and 3) testimonial incompetence must follow from, or appear to follow from, pernicious ignorance.   (2011: 244)

Although the speaker in a case of testimonial smothering cuts short *her own* testimony, doing so is coerced or forced upon her by features of the situation. The notion of 'unsafe and risky' testimony refers to the idea that harm or negative effects could follow. In the context of a contact-tracing interview, divulging certain information might feed into negative stereotypes about the group the individual is from (e.g., someone might not disclose that they had a drink with a friend at a bar if they are from a group often disparagingly associated with alcoholism). This might be particularly likely if there is an expectation that the contact tracer might not be able to accurately assess the truth of the testimony. For instance, someone who has previously had their symptoms unfairly dismissed by a health professional may expect other health professionals, including the public health officials involved in contact tracing, to be similarly unable to competently assess her testimony. It would meet the third condition if the speaker's assessment of the contact tracer's (in)competence was informed by some racist or classist comment or act which primes the speaker to believe that the contact tracer does not believe her or does not make an effort to understand or evaluate her testimony.

## Trust, Fairness, and Knowledge in Public Health Emergencies

Cases of epistemic injustice and testimonial smothering prompt questions about the trust relationships between individuals from marginalized or oppressed social groups, and the authority figures engaged in managing public health emergencies. In this final section of the paper we argue that distrust can be mutual in these cases, and that it can give rise to dysfunctional epistemic practices which *both* fail to achieve knowledge goals *and* perpetuate injustice.

Trust, following Annette Baier (1986), is an attitude moral agents have towards one another, typically accompanied by normatively laden expectations that the trusted person will show good will rather than ill will. The disappointment of trust generally results in negative morally reactive attitudes, such as resentment, anger, or a sense of betrayal. Baier distinguishes trust from mere reliance. Reliance involves depending on people or things without making normative attributions if the expectation is not met. Thus, one may trust the doctor to act on a principle of beneficence, but merely rely on a tennis ball to bounce.

Baier draws attention to the involvement of power in trust interactions. The person who trusts is vulnerable to the trusted person. But where there is already a power inequity this relationship can become distorted. These include cases 'where the truster relies on his threat advantage to keep the trust relation going' (Baier 1986: 255).

Baier does not focus on the connections between trust and epistemology or epistemic injustice, but other philosophers do. Both Katherine Hawley (2017) and Jose Medina (2020) note that trust has a sincerity and competence dimension. The trusted person is only trustworthy if she is both competent to deliver the trusted testimony or action, and sincerely intends to do so (and not, for example, mislead or betray). Hawley regards only the competence dimension as epistemic, arguing that wrongly judging someone to be insincere does not harm them in their capacity as a knower, but wrongly judging their testimony to be incompetent does.

Members of disadvantaged groups have significant historical basis for distrusting public health officials. In the United States, the Tuskagee Syphilis Study is a well-known case in which public health research into the natural course of untreated syphilis was allowed to run in an African American population until 1972 despite the emergence of penicillin as an effective and widely available treatment during this time. The researchers harmed the study participants, deceived them, and deliberately withheld gold standard treatment (Brandt 1978). More recently, in the aftermath of Hurricane Katrina in New Orleans, African Americans perceived racism in multiple aspects of the handling of the emergency. This included support and processes for evacuation of the city; speed of response in the aftermath, and descriptions of white Americans as 'finding' food as opposed to African Americans as 'looting' (Blodorn et al. 2016).

This distrust may increase the likelihood of testimonial smothering, which (as described in the previous section) might frustrate public health efforts. Where a positive case is not forthcoming with their movements to contact tracers, this very silence might be risky for the marginalized group, reinforcing a prejudiced perception of members of that group as uncooperative. One potential consequence of this is the imposition of more extreme surveillance measures.

In New South Wales during the 2021 Covid-19 Delta outbreak, something like this appeared to happen. The outbreak began in the wealthy area of Bondi Beach and surrounds, and rapidly spread. Within weeks, case numbers started to increase in poorer areas in the south-west of Sydney, where a higher percentage of the population are immigrants.

It was when the outbreak became established in these poorer areas with large migrant populations that public health officials recommended more intrusive forms of surveillance. Moreover, some measures were only implemented in specific suburbs—often suburbs with significant socially marginalized or disadvantaged populations. These surveillance mechanisms included mandatory surveillance testing of all workers who needed to leave the area to work. Arguably, these measures reflected credibility deficits or distrust towards this community—certainly some perceived this to be the case, although it was denied by officials. The sense that the local surveillance measures reflected distrust by the authorities was reinforced when the authorities did not impose the same measures on residents of the wealthy Bondi area where the outbreak emerged.

Alongside increased public health surveillance measures—such as mandatory testing—are surveillance and other activities aimed at enforcement of public health orders. The use of numberplate scanning, increased police presence, and military involvement in the poorer suburbs in the southwest of Sydney increased perceptions of racism and classism in the public health response. This, in turn, contributed to knowledge-related dysfunction. Protests against public health orders (including vaccination programs and mandatory face masks) indicated failures of knowledge sharing, failures of (some) citizens to extend epistemic trust to authorities, and threatened the effectiveness of the public health response. According to Baier's account of trust, it can be morally bad or corrupt to maintain trust in someone who has been deceiving or coercing you in past trust situations (Baier 1986). Thus, oppressed groups' distrust in public health officials may be morally warranted, placing the onus on the public health officials to break the vicious cycle.

## Conclusion

In this chapter, we have outlined some key features of public health emergencies and outlined epistemic features associated with surveillance. Drawing on a case study of the New South Wales response to the 2021 Covid-19 Delta outbreak, we argued that some of these features contribute to risks of epistemic injustice and dysfunctions of trust. These, in turn, can threaten the knowledge-related goals of surveillance as well as potentially undermining the effectiveness of the public health response to the emergency. For this reason, officials cannot consider the knowledge-related goals of surveillance in public health emergencies without considering (and attempting to mitigate) any associated risks of epistemic injustice and dysfunctions of trust.

## References

Asghar H., Diop O. M., Weldegebriel G., Malik F., Shetty S., El Bassioni L., Akande A. O., Al Maamoun E., Zaidi S., Adeniji A. J., Burns C. C. 2014. 'Environmental surveillance for polioviruses in the Global Polio Eradication Initiative'. *The Journal of infectious diseases*. 210 (suppl_1) (Nov 1): S294–303.

Baier A. 1986. 'Trust and Antitrust'. *Ethics* 96 (2) (1 Jan): 231–60.

Blakely, B., Rogers, W., Johnson, J. *et al.* Ethical and regulatory implications of the COVID-19 pandemic for the medical devices industry and its representatives. *BMC Med Ethics* 23, 31 (2022).

Blodorn A, O'Brien LT, Cheryan S, Vick SB. Understanding perceptions of racism in the aftermath of hurricane Katrina: The roles of system and group justification. *Social Justice Research.* 2016 Jun; 29(2):139–58.

Bouri N. and Ravi, S. 2014. 'Going Mobile: How Mobile Personal Health Records Can Improve Health Care during Emergencies'. *JMIR mHealth and uHealth* 2 (1) (5 Mar): e3017.

Brandt, A. M. 1978. 'Racism and Research: The Case of the Tuskegee Syphilis Study'. *Hastings Center Report* (1 Dec): 21–9.

Calderwood, Kathleen. 2021. "CCTV Captures 'scarily Fleeting' Encounter That Resulting in Bondi COVID-19 Cluster Growing." *ABC News*, June 21, 2021. https://www.abc.net.au/news/2021-06-22/covid19-cctv-footage-worrying-nsw-health-authorities/100231832.

Canali, S. 2016. 'Big Data, Epistemology and Causality: Knowledge in and Knowledge Out in EXPOsOMICS'. *Big Data & Society* 3 (2) (Sept): 2053951716669530.

Conifer, Dan. 2021. "The COVIDSafe App Has Cost $9m to Date, but It Hasn't Uncovered Any Close Contacts during the Current Outbreaks." *ABC News*, September 30, 2021. https://www.abc.net.au/news/2021-09-30/covidsafe-app-cost-hasnt-uncovered-close-contacts-2021-outbreaks/100499870.

Curtis, Katina, and Rachel Clun. 2020. "Card Payment Data to Be Used to Track People in Coronavirus Hotspots." The Sydney Morning Herald. November 13, 2020. https://www.smh.com.au/politics/federal/card-payment-data-to-be-used-to-track-people-in-coronavirus-hotspots-20201113-p56eea.html.

Degeling C., Hall J., Johnson J., Abbas R., Bag S., and Gilbert, G. L. 2021. 'Should Digital Contact Tracing Technologies be used to Control COVID-19? Perspectives from an Australian Public Deliberation'. *Health Care Analysis* 26 (Oct): 1–8.

Dotson, K. 2011. 'Tracking Epistemic Violence, Tracking Practices of Silencing'. *Hypatia* 26 (2): 236–57.

Foege, W. H., Hogan, R. C., and Newton, L. H. 1976. 'Surveillance Projects for Selected Diseases'. *International Journal of Epidemiology* 5 (1) (1 Mar): 29–37.

Frické, M. 2015. 'Big Data and Its Epistemology'. *Journal of the Association for Information Science and Technology* 66 (4) (Apr): 651–61. https://asistdl.onlinelibrary.wiley.com/doi/abs/10.1002/asi.23212

Fricker, M. 2007. *Epistemic Injustice: Power and the Ethics of Knowing.* Oxford: Oxford University Press.

Hanrahan, Catherine. 2021. "How Your Phone, and Tech Giants Google and Facebook, Helped Shape NSW's Pandemic Response." *ABC News*, October 19, 2021. https://www.abc.net.au/news/2021-10-20/tech-giants-tracing-helped-predict-covid-peaks/100550964.

Hawley, K. J. 2017. 'Trust, Distrust and Epistemic Injustice'. In *Routledge Handbook of Epistemic Injustice*, edited by I. J. Kidd, J. Medina, and G. Pohlhaus. Abingdon and New York: Routledge.

Health Protection NSW. 2023. "COVID-19 Sewage Surveillance Program - COVID-19 (Coronavirus)." January 19, 2023. https://www.health.nsw.gov.au:443/Infectious/covid-19/Pages/sewage-surveillance.aspx.

Housen, Tambri. 2020. "What Can You Expect If You Get a Call from a COVID Contact Tracer?" The Conversation. November 26, 2020. http://theconversation.com/what-can-you-expect-if-you-get-a-call-from-a-covid-contact-tracer-150742.

Housen, T. What Can You Expect If You Get a Call from a COVID Contact Tracer?' *The Conversation*, 26 November 2020. Online at https://theconversation.com/what-can-you-expect-if-you-get-a-call-from-a-covid-contact-tracer-150742

Irmiter, C., Subbarao, I., Shah, J. N., Sokol, P., and James, J. J. 2012. 'Personal Derived Health Information: A Foundation to Preparing the United States for Disasters and Public Health Emergencies'. *Disaster Medicine and Public Health Preparedness* 6 (3) (Oct): 303–10.

Johnson, I., Hansen, A., and Bi, P. 2018. 'The Challenges of Implementing an Integrated One Health Surveillance System in Australia'. *Zoonoses and Public Health* 65 (1) (Feb): e229–36. https://onlinelibrary.wiley.com/doi/full/10.1111/zph.12433

Johnson, J., Howard, K., Wilson, A., Ward, M., Gilbert, G. L., and Degeling, C. 2019. 'Public Preferences for One Health Approaches to Emerging Infectious Diseases: A Discrete Choice Experiment'. *Social Science & Medicine* 228 (1 May): 164–71.

Kupersmith, J., Francis, J., Kerr, E., Krein, S., Pogach, L., Kolodner, R. M., and Perlin, J. B. 2007. 'Advancing Evidence-Based Care For Diabetes: Lessons From The Veterans Health Administration: A Highly Regarded EHR System Is but One Contributor to the Quality Transformation of the VHA since the mid-1990s'. *Health Affairs* 26 (Suppl1): w156–68.

Lamarche-Vadel, A., Pavillon, G., Aouba, A., Johansson, L. A., Meyer, L., Jougla, E., Rey, G. 2014. 'Automated Comparison of Last Hospital Main Diagnosis and Underlying Cause of Death ICD10 Codes, France, 2008–2009'. *BMC Medical Informatics and Decision Making* 14 (1) (Dec): 1–9.

Leonelli, S. 2014. 'What Difference Does Quantity Make? On the Epistemology of Big Data in Biology'. *Big Data & Society* 1 (1) (10 July): 2053951714534395.

Lipworth, W., Mason, P. H., Kerridge, I., Ioannidis, J. P. 2017. 'Ethics and Epistemology in Big Data Research'. *Journal of Bioethical Inquiry* 14 (4) (Dec): 489–500.

Mazzocchi, F. 2015. 'Could Big Data Be the End of Theory in Science? A Few Remarks on the Epistemology of Data-Driven Science'. *EMBO Reports* 16 (10) (Oct): 1250–5.

Medina, J. 2020. 'Trust and Epistemic Injustice'. In *The Routledge Handbook of Trust and Philosophy*, edited by J. Simon, 52–63. Abingdon and New York: Routledge.

Melnick J. L. 1947. 'Poliomyelitis Virus in Urban Sewage in Epidemic and in Nonepidemic Times'. *American journal of hygiene.* 45 (2): 240–53.

Moe K. 1984. 'Should the Nazi research data be cited?' *Hastings Center Report*. 14 (6) (Dec): 5–7.

Murdoch, T. B. and Detsky, A. S. 2013. 'The Inevitable Application of Big Data to Health Care'. *JAMA* 309 (13) (3 Apr): 1351–2.

Nevo, I. Y. 2010. 'The Makings of Good Science: Epistemology and Ethics'. *Israel Journal of Ecology and Evolution* 57 (4) (6 May): 319–30.

Nsubuga, P., White, M. E., Thacker, S. B., Anderson, M. A., Blount, S. B., Broome, C. V., Chiller, T. M., Espitia, V., Imtiaz, R., Sosin, D., and Stroup, D. F. 2006. 'Public Health Surveillance: A Tool for Targeting and Monitoring Interventions'. In *Disease Control Priorities in Developing Countries*, 2nd edn, edited by D. T. Jamison, J. G. Breman, A. R. Measham et al. https://www.ncbi.nlm.nih.gov/books/NBK11770/

Porsdam Mann, S., Savulescu, J., and Sahakian, B. J. 2016. 'Facilitating the Ethical Use of Health Data for the Benefit of Society: Electronic Health Records, Consent and the Duty of Easy Rescue'. *Philosophical Transactions of the Royal Society A: Mathematical, Physical and Engineering Sciences* 374 (2083) (28 Dec): 20160130.

Post, S. G. 1991. 'The Echo of Nuremberg: Nazi Data and Ethics'. *Journal of Medical Ethics* 17 (1) (1 Mar): 42–4.

Samerski, S. 2018. 'Individuals on Alert: Digital Epidemiology and the Individualization of Surveillance'. *Life Sciences, Society and Policy* 14 (1) (Dec): 1–1.

Thackway, S., Churches, T., Fizzell, J., Muscatello, D., and Armstrong, P. 2009. 'Should Alert: Digital Epidemiology and the Individualization of Surveillance. *BMC Public Health* 9 (1) (Dec): 1–0.

Tu, J. V., Chu, A., Donovan, L. R., Ko, D. T., Booth, G. L., Tu, K., Maclagan, L. C., Guo, H., Austin, P. C., Hogg, W., and Kapral, M. K. 2015. 'The Cardiovascular Health in Ambulatory Care Research Team (CANHEART) Using Big Data to Measure and Improve Cardiovascular Health and Healthcare Services'. *Circulation: Cardiovascular Quality and Outcomes* 8 (2) (Mar): 204–12.

Tuvel, R. 2015. Against the Use of Knowledge Gained from Animal Experimentation'. *Societies* 5 (1) (Mar): 220–44.

Yee, A., Zubovic, E., Yu, J., Ray, S., Hildebrandt, S., Seidelman, W. E., Polak, R. J., Grodin, M. A., Coert, J. H., Brown, D., Kodner, I. J. 2009. 'Ethical Considerations in the Use of Pernkopf's Atlas of Anatomy: A Surgical Case Study'. *Surgery* 165 (5) (1 May): 860–7.

World Health Organization. 2016. International Health Regulations (2005), 3rd edn. http://www.who.int/ihr/publications/9789241580496/en/

# PART II
# ETHICS IN TIMES OF
# EMERGENCY

# 6

# Surveillance without 'Baddies'

## Liability and Consent in Non-Antagonistic Surveillance Ethics

*Kasper Lippert-Rasmussen and Kira Vrist Rønn*

According to one influential definition, surveillance is 'any systematic and routine attention to personal details, whether specific or aggregate, for a defined purpose' (Lyon 2014: 2). Most theorists assume that surveillance, so defined, is morally problematic when it is non-consensual, e.g., because of how it violates privacy rights. For present purposes, we shall simply assume that non-consensual surveillance is morally problematic. However, whether this is the case—and if so, why—is a huge question in itself.[1]

The majority of scholars exploring the ethics of surveillance primarily address the issue in antagonistic contexts—roughly, contexts in which a wrongful aggressor intends to harm or wrong an innocent victim, and a rightful defender surveils the aggressor to prevent the harm or wrong. Examples of such contexts include counter-terrorism and crime prevention/crime detection (Kleinig 2009; Lyon 2014; Macnish 2014, 2015; Marx 1998). Accordingly, many scholars have drawn on distinctions from the ethics of war and self-defence in order to develop a framework for surveillance ethics (Bellaby 2012; Kleinig 2009; Macnish 2014, 2015; Nathan 2017; Rønn and Lippert-Rasmussen 2020).[2] Such frameworks naturally focus on considerations regarding the *liability* of the surveilled and how it affects the moral permissibility of surveillance.

---

[1] First, theorists distinguish between *bodily privacy* and *informational privacy* (Solove 2008; Tavani 2008). Second, surveillance scholars distinguish between informational privacy violations as being a question of either *loss of control* of private information or someone *accessing* this information for a defined purpose (Macnish 2018). Third, scholarship specifies different forms of 'bads' and 'wrongs' related to surveillance, e.g., the loss of freedom and the (potential) abuse of power that is facilitated by collecting and storing citizens' (personal) information (in democratic societies) (Stahl 2016). For present purposes, we need not go into the complications raised by these three distinctions, since whichever aspect of privacy or harm one focuses on, pandemic-related surveillance may infringe such aspects of privacy, and give rise to relevant kinds of harm. However, not all uses of Covid-19 tracking apps violate privacy rights (however construed) (see section: 'Why Consent Might Matter').
[2] Some scholars are sceptical about transferring the distinctions from the ethical theories on self-defence and just war to surveillance (see, e.g. Diderichsen and Rønn 2017; Lever 2016; Stoddart 2014). It is beyond the scope of this chapter to address this scepticism.

Kasper Lippert-Rasmussen and Kira Vrist Rønn, *Surveillance without 'Baddies': Liability and Consent in Non-Antagonistic Surveillance Ethics* In: *The Ethics of Surveillance in Times of Emergency*. Edited by: Kevin Macnish and Adam Henschke, Oxford University Press. © Oxford University Press 2023. DOI: 10.1093/oso/9780192864918.003.0007

The Coronavirus pandemic, which presents a potentially lethal threat to the affected individuals, motivates broadening the focus of the ethics of surveillance to non-antagonistic contexts. The reason for this is that one way of reducing the spread of Covid-19 is through the use of various surveillance methods. In this chapter, we will focus on the use of Covid-19 tracking apps or, more generally, infection tracking apps. While Covid-19 is the first occasion on which such surveillance devices have received significant attention, other pandemics or more run-of-the-mill infections, e.g., the common flu, raise essentially the same issues as the Covid-19 pandemic, though the stakes might typically be lower or unfortunately, in some future pandemics, higher. Such apps are intended to warn people against close contact with infected individuals, facilitate identification of anyone who has been in contact with somebody infected, and ensure appropriate testing and self-isolation (Stanley and Granick 2020). Many different versions of such apps exist, and the risks related to these innovations vary depending on the specific design concerned.[3]

In infection-related surveillance contexts, there is no human *aggressor* and, therefore, no antagonistic relationship between *the surveillant* and *the surveilled*. Accordingly, many might find it unclear that anyone is liable to any form of intervention that, in the absence of actions for which they are responsible, would constitute a wrongful intervention against them. Accordingly, in the next section, we address the question of whether and in what form liability plays a role in surveillance ethics in the context of pandemics. Can persons who are not responsible for catching an infectious disease, and who do not intend to harm or wrong others by transmitting it, be liable to surveillance because they pose a threat? If so, are they innocent or culpable threats? We argue that infection-bearers—and, for that matter, people who think that they might be bearers of an infection, but in fact are not—can very easily become liable threats by failing to minimize the risk they pose to others. In failing to do so, they become culpable threats and, therefore, liable to certain forms of intervention that would otherwise wrong them. We refer to these as *negligent, liable threats*. We focus on liability to surveillance through infection-tracking apps. However, tracking apps in themselves might do little to mitigate epidemics. People need to act on the information obtained by such devices, e.g., by taking a test and by self-isolating if the test is positive. If they do not take such steps voluntarily, in our view they might become

---

[3] In general, a core distinction between the types of infection-tracking apps is whether they store all collected information on citizens' movements and infection status in a central register or in decentralized locations, only accessible to individual phone users. The centralized version enables the authorities to follow closely both the development in infection rates and the attitude and behaviour of citizens (Stanley and Granick 2020). It also enables a type and range of surveillance that is unfamiliar in democratic societies and creates a significant vulnerability, namely the risk of hacking of such registers and misuse at the hands of the authorities (Stahl 2016). Many liberal democracies have opted for the decentralized version. In this chapter, we focus our attention on the use of tracking apps in liberal societies, where the risk of information being misused is relatively low.

liable to involuntary testing or quarantine. We believe liability extend to such measures as well in case they are not taken voluntarily.

Our argument in the third section raises the question of the moral significance of consent in relation to infection-related surveillance. In this context, however, a dilemma might easily arise. On the one hand, the developers and health authorities in many countries emphasize that *consent* on the part of the users of Covid-19 related apps is a crucial concern. On the other hand, widespread use of the app—and, of course, appropriate precautionary measure typically being taken in response to the information being provided through the apps—is necessary to achieve the desired effect (according to Oxford researchers, around 80 per cent of the population should download the app) (Vaughan 2020), yet such levels of usage are unlikely to be achieved if consent is required.

The third section argues that the alleged trade-off between the effectiveness of surveillance-based means of fighting infections—or, more generally, non-antagonistic surveillance contexts—on the one hand, and accommodating concern for people's consent on the other, is much less of a dilemma than it might otherwise have been. This assumes that many, if not most, who do not use infection tracing apps are culpable threats. As such, these people are not wronged by surveillance measures being imposed upon them, regardless of whether they consent to these measures.[4]

The third section might give the impression that we think that, morally speaking, there is no reason to favour voluntary infection surveillance measures over non- or involuntary surveillance measures, or that consent to surveillance is morally irrelevant. The penultimate section cautions against this impression in two ways. First, it argues that offering the surveilled the option to consent can make a difference to what it is possible to do to the surveilled without wronging them. Second, even setting aside considerations about wronging, offering citizens the option to consent might have inherent moral value. In relation to discussions of the morality of paternalism, it is generally thought that paternalistic policies are disrespectful because they send the message that the state deems citizens incapable of doing what is best for themselves, or at least unlikely to do so. We argue that if that is the case, then the state similarly treats citizens disrespectfully by not offering them the option of consenting to infection related surveillance, and by sending the message that they are incapable of making the morally right choice, or

---

[4] Jeff McMahan (2009: 159) defines culpable threats as 'people who pose a threat of wrongful harm to others and have neither justification, permission, nor excuse'. Also, according to McMahan's (2009: 10) account, people are liable to attack, or other unwanted interventions, when the circumstances dictate that they have forfeited their rights not to be subjected to this treatment. One can be liable without culpability, e.g., if one innocently poses a threat of wrongful harm to others, as in McMahan's (2009: 165) example of the conscientious driver whose car unpredictably veers out of control and towards a pedestrian.

at least unlikely to do so. This might not amount to wronging citizens, but it might still be morally unjustified.

The final section briefly concludes by summing up our main claims regarding the moral justifiability of infection tracking apps in general, and Covid-19 tracking apps specifically.


## Liability of (Potential) Infection Bearers

As already noted, many discussions of the ethics of surveillance draw on the ethics of war and self-defence. The paradigmatic case that such ethical theories address is one in which an aggressor (a state or an individual) wrongfully attacks a defender (another state or individual). Most agree that in such cases, the defender is morally permitted to do things to the aggressor that, in the absence of the aggression, would have wronged the aggressor, notably using lethal force to thwart the attack. One central explanation of why this is morally permissible is that the aggressor poses an unjust threat, and thus has become liable to defensive force (Clark 2000; Uniacke 2011). The aggressor has unjustly made it the case that, unavoidably, someone or other will suffer harm, and justice requires that this harm befalls the aggressor who made it unavoidable, rather than someone else. This means that the aggressor's rights, e.g., to life, are not violated when the aggressor is killed in proportionate self-defence and has no moral complaint against the defender's use of lethal force against them. Alternatively, if the defender could save their life by attacking an innocent bystander, this would not be permissible. An innocent bystander does not pose any threat to the defender and is therefore not liable to the use of any force (McMahan 1994; 2009). Hence, liability is crucial to the principle of discrimination, i.e., that lethal (or at least severely harmful) force can only be used against aggressors/combatants, and not against bystanders/civilians.[5]

If we move from the context of war and physical aggression to surveillance in counter-terrorism or crime prevention/crime detection, i.e., what we have referred to as antagonistic settings, it seems natural to assume that liability plays a similarly crucial role (Nathan 2017; Macnish 2015). Following McMahan, we assume that a person is liable to defensive harm if, and only if, he or she morally responsible for posing an objectively unjustified threat. Something resembling the principle of discrimination naturally applies to surveillance, too. In other words, there is a crucial difference between how, say, people who are (reasonably suspected of

---

[5] Liability is also central to the principle of proportionality. Theories of just war and self-defence generally assume that the use of force must be proportional. This means that the balance between the inflicted harms and the severity of the infringements in question, on the one hand, and the anticipated benefits, on the other, must be sufficiently favourable for the use of force to be justified.

being) terrorists or organized criminals might be surveilled, and how ordinary citizens might be surveilled, since, arguably, only the former are liable to surveillance (Nathan 2017; Rønn and Lippert-Rasmussen 2020; Stahl 2016). Similarly, liability also plays a crucial role in determining whether surveillance is proportionate (Kleinig 2009; Macnish 2014, 2015, 2018; Marx 1998; Nathan 2017, Rønn and Lippert-Rasmussen 2020). As with theories of just war and self-defence, it is the norm to distinguish between narrow proportionality (cases in which surveillance is directed intentionally at liable threats) and wide proportionality (cases in which surveillance is intentionally or unintentionally directed towards non-liable threats), and then focus on the former (McMahan 2009; Rønn and Lippert-Rasmussen 2020). Hence, liability is also central to surveillance ethics (cp. Diderichsen and Rønn 2017).

Turning now to surveillance in the context of infections and surveillance, some might find the idea that liability plays a significant role strange. The reason for this is not that, offhand, liability appears never applicable to this context. If I deliberately infect myself with, say, Covid-19 and seek to transmit the disease to as many vulnerable people as possible by deliberately coughing on them, it is natural to say that I am liable to surveillance (and even to harsher measures such as quarantine). However, the point is that generally speaking, hardly anyone would appear to be liable for Covid-19-related reasons. Unlike in our previous example, people are not, on the whole, morally responsible for becoming bearers of the disease—quite the contrary—and people do not generally seek to transmit the disease to others. Hence, in practice, it might seem that the distinction between liable and non-liable is largely irrelevant to Covid-19-related surveillance, as virtually everyone is non-liable.

However, this initial view is problematic. There are at least three ways to reach that conclusion. First, there is the straightforward observation that many people are in fact responsible for acting in ways which impose, and they are aware impose, a significant risk on others of transmitting the disease to them, e.g., by attending large gatherings or by refusing to wear masks and then interacting with others. Such behaviour plausibly gives rise to liability to modest interventions to prevent people from transmitting the relevant disease.[6]

Second, consider Robert Nozick's classic discussion of *innocent threats*. He imagines a person who is unexpectedly caught by a gust of wind and hurled down a well. At the bottom of the well is another person, who will be crushed to death when the falling person lands. The falling person, however, will survive unharmed. According to Nozick and many others, the person at the bottom of the well could

---

[6] There is a moral difference between liable to lethal force and liability to surveillance through infection apps in that, intuitively, more is required for liability to the former than to the latter much less harmful intervention.

shoot the innocent threat without violating the falling person's rights if doing so would somehow save their own life (Nozick 1974: 34).[7] One view here is that in this case, the innocent threat is liable to defensive harm, since the person at the bottom of the well has a right not to be killed. This right is infringed by the falling person, whose falling body is causally responsible for the threat to the person in the well (Thomson 1991). This is so even if the falling person is in no way morally responsible for his falling body posing a deadly threat to the person at the bottom of the well.

Many will find it highly implausible that facts for which individuals bear no moral responsibility can render them liable to deadly defensive force (Clark 2000). Still, if we accept this view—and some will argue that we must in order to be able to explain why it is morally permissible for the person at the bottom of the well to defend themselves—then a similar view applies in the case of infection-related surveillance. A person who is innocently unaware that she might infect others because she is innocently unaware of both the fact that she has Covid-19 and the fact that, relative to what she knows, she might infect others with Covid-19, is an innocent threat to others in much the same way as Nozick's person who is picked up by the wind and thrown into a well (Lippert-Rasmussen 2020). If we agree that we do, in fact, all pose innocent threats to others, since we could all potentially be infected with Covid-19, are we then allowed to infringe on, e.g., others' rights to privacy or other freedoms as self-defence against a morally innocent, but liable, threat? For instance, would it be possible to forcibly install tracking apps on smartphones without wrongfully violating the users' rights?[8] If we accept the analogy of the falling person in Nozick's example, the answer would be yes. Hence, we might reframe the analogy in the context of Covid-19, and claim that we all have a right not to be infected by others, and therefore it is permissible to infringe another person's (and our own) rights, e.g., the right to privacy, as an act of self-defence against the innocent but rights-violating threat that we all pose.

Some may find this line of reasoning problematic. For example, McMahan argues against the conclusion of the falling person example, asserting that 'a

---

[7] For reasons of space, we ignore the distinction between fact-relative and evidence-relative threats. If X aims an unloaded gun at you with the apparent intention of pulling the trigger, X is an evidence-relative threat (from your perspective), even if they are not one in the fact-relative sense. Since virtually all of us could be infected with Covid-19, virtually all of us are evidence-relative threats to others. We have slightly modified Nozick's original example, in which it is a villain who throws the bystander into the well, to avoid the moral complication to which the presence of a culpable human agent gives rise. Thomson exemplifies a similar point in a slightly different way. In her example, *the falling man*, a man is having a picnic on a cliff just above you (and unluckily, you cannot move, because your leg is stuck). A third person pushes the picnicking man off the cliff, and his fall will be lethal for you, but the man will survive. However, you can choose to unfold your umbrella, impale the falling man and survive (Thomson 1991).

[8] As an anonymous reviewer pointed out, governments might not even need to go this far. They could demand the data from the mobile phone companies, giving precise location of the phone at all times, thus, providing useful information for identifying and stopping disease transmission chains.

person cannot be morally constrained from being involuntarily acted upon by physical forces' (McMahan 2009: 388). However, others might not find this exchange particularly relevant, on the grounds that when it comes to Covid-19, most of us are not *innocent* threats to others. This is where the second argument to which we referred comes into play.

Consider a person who acts in a way that results in a significantly heightened risk that he or she might pass on the disease to others, e.g., because she refrains from installing a Covid-19 tracking device on her smartphone despite interacting with others in ways where she could transmit Covid-19 to them.[9] True, such a person is different from the paradigmatic aggressor in theories of just war and self-defence in that they do not *aim* to harm or wrong others. However, this might simply show that a threat can be non-innocent, and therefore liable to defensive force for reasons other than those at play in the paradigmatic cases of just war and self-defence theories. More specifically, it shows that an individual can become liable to defensive force through *negligence* (see McMahan 2009: 160).

Negligence can take many forms. The relevant form here seems to amount to an inappropriately limited concern for the vital interests of others, in order to avoid what is at most a rather minor setback of the individual's own non-vital interests. A person who refuses to install an infection-tracing app is perhaps a bit like one refusing to quarantine when told to and, therefore, knowingly exposing many others to the risk of infection. Or, to elaborate upon Nozick's well-known example, they are like a person who negligently ventures outside for no particular reason and refuses to download a 'wind gust-meter' on their smartphone that would prevent them from being turned into a human projectile and posing a risk to others.

At this point, some might object that it is somewhat ad hoc to claim that negligence can render the individual liable to the use of self-defensive force, even rather mild forms of self-defensive force, such as the compulsory installation of an infection-tracking app on a smartphone or compulsory test and self-isolation in relation to an infection-tracking app detection of a high risk of infection. However, this worry is ungrounded. In just war theory, a country can be a just

---

[9] While one can be liable to surveillance for reasons not having to do with the omission to download a tracking app, our view is that one's omission to do so is itself a source of liability and a factor that affects the degree of forceful intervention that one becomes liable to (see the discussion in the section on 'Consent of Liable Bearers of Infectious Diseases'). In a discussion of McMahan's view that a conscientious driver who is responsible for posing a threat to a pedestrian he is about to run down as a result of an unpredictable mechanical malfunction is liable to defensive force (see footnote 4). Quong (2020: 35) suggests, pace McMahan, that conscientious driving does not make on liable to defensive force, because the practice of driving is an advantage to everyone and is morally permissible despite the known fact that each year a number of pedestrians will be run down accidentally. This view applied to infections would imply that one does not become liable simply by interacting with others, thus, imposing a risk on a lethal infection on them. However, Quong's view would not apply to interacting with others without an infection tracking device, provided that this is an effective and costless way of avoiding imposing risk on others.

aggressor through negligence, e.g., by omitting to take proper precautions against accidentally launching missiles. Similarly, in theories of self-defence, if I start firing a gun in the direction of a bunch of innocent people—not to harm them, but simply to check whether the gun works—I become liable to defensive force intended to prevent the threat that I myself pose negligently. Indeed, this defensive force may be just as severe as it would be had I shot at them with the intention to kill.

Suppose that negligence can render people liable to the use of defensive force. This might not be particularly relevant to Covid-19-related surveillance if few of us ever negligently expose others to the risk of our transmitting the disease to them, or if the defensive measures in question were disproportionate. However, none of these suppositions seems true. First, we conjecture that most people at least occasionally interact with others while failing to observe the rules of social distancing, handwashing, etc., and know that they do so.[10] In addition, many people might negligently put themselves in a position where they risk being infected, e.g., by attending large gatherings (WHO 2020). In itself, this might not make them liable to any defensive measures. However, it might if, at the same time, they engage in behaviour that means they risk transmitting the disease to others. Second, the defensive measures in question—e.g., downloading a tracing app, submitting to a test if the app detects a high risk of having contracted the infection, and compulsory self-isolation for one or two weeks if the test is positive—are quite modest ones (in democracies at least, where risks of state of abuse are relatively minor) compared to the defensive measures normally justified in theories of just war and self-defence and in the light of the risks involved in contracting serious infections such as Covid-19. Naturally, being liable does not imply a *carte-blanche* for infection-related right-infringements. However, it will justify some forms of morally permissible (self-)defence against further infection, e.g., mandatory self-isolation. In this context, downloading a tracking app seems like a relatively easily justifiable intervention.

In the light of the above, we are inclined to infer that many of us, if not most of us, are indeed negligently exposing others to a risk of contagion. It therefore seems relevant, for a wide range of cases, to approach the issue of infection-related surveillance via the lens of just war and self-defence theory. If this is correct, it raises an important question about the significance of consent in connection with infection-related surveillance, which we will address in the following section.

---

[10] Admittedly, some people might be innocent threats. The exact number depends on the threshold required for innocence—e.g., whether an individual who acts according to official guidelines is a non-responsible threat, who arguably would be wronged if others intervened to prevent them from spreading Covid-19.

## Consent of Liable Bearers of Infectious Diseases
## and Tracing Apps

Infection-tracking smartphone apps, which are intended to inform citizens about contact with infected persons, are one of the most common and widespread surveillance initiatives in the context of Covid-19 (Stanley and Granick 2020).

The developers and health agencies in many European countries attach great value to smartphone holders consenting to the use of these apps. However, developers and users in other countries attach less significance to whether users provide valid consent. For instance, in some countries, the state makes it impossible for citizens to perform certain acts that entail a risk of contagion, e.g., buying a train ticket, if they don't have the app on their smartphone or if the app classifies them as likely carriers of Covid-19 (see e.g., Dukakis 2020). If you're treated for Covid-19, healthcare authorities confiscate your smartphone and enter information regarding your health status. They even use the information provided by your app to identify and contact those with whom you have had contact, to force *them* to take a Covid-19 test. In the light of our discussion in the second section, the following question arises: does the consent-centric approach attach too much moral significance to valid consent on the part of users of Covid-19 tracking apps?

To see why this question is relevant, we must return to the ethics of war and self-defence. In this context, we argued that non-innocent, negligent threats are liable to defensive force and that most of us are negligent threats to others.[11] If this view is correct, then a corollary seems to be that there is no moral requirement that non-innocent threats consent to their being exposed to defensive force. The reason for this is that generally speaking, we do not have the right to refuse the imposition upon us of relatively minor forms of harm, etc., to prevent us from transmitting serious infections to others, which we have the moral power to relinquish. A crucial element that enables the possibility of giving normatively valid consent is missing. Consider a relevant and similar example from the ethics of self-defence. If I start firing a gun in your direction, with the aim of testing whether it works, you do not need my consent to tamper with my smartphone if that would somehow prevent you from being negligently shot by me. You do not even need my consent before it is permissible to return fire. Similarly, if I regularly venture out, despite having symptoms that could be indicative of Covid-19, or despite having recently been with others who have visited areas with high levels of contagion, then I impose a significant risk on you of contracting Covid-19. In that case, you do not need my consent to tamper with my smartphone to install a tracking device. Nor, if the tracking device indicates high risk of infection and you

---

[11] We also mentioned that according to some views, even non-innocent threats might be liable to defensive force. We are sceptical of this view. However, note that if it is correct, then that strengthens our scepticism about the significance of consent.

persist in imposing a high risk on others which they cannot avoid or can avoid only at great cost to themselves, do you need my consent to a quick test and, if the test is positive, to quarantine me for a limited period of time, if doing so would somehow significantly reduce your risk of getting infected with a potentially lethal virus.[12]

If we say that consent is not morally required for the negligent threat not to be wronged by the imposition of defensive force, that is not to say that there is no moral significance in the negligent threat accepting such an imposition. Let us consider a standard example in the ethics of self-defence. If, say, the negligent shooter has consented in advance to being subjected to defensive force should they negligently start firing their gun in the direction of innocent people, then, plausibly, the fact that subjecting the negligent shooter to defensive force will harm them constitutes even less of a moral objection to defending yourself against the negligent threat. Similarly, the view defended here is consistent with saying that while it is not morally required to obtain the consent of negligent potential bearers of Covid-19, the fact that they consent lessens any moral objection to them being subjected to Covid-19-related surveillance.[13]

In fact, if people have the option to consent to download a Covid-19 tracking app, then not consenting is arguably morally significant in a different way.[14] To refuse to consent to download it, when you reasonably believe that you might impose a risk on others of contracting the disease, could in itself constitute a form of morally objectionable negligence.[15] After all, you are provided with a relatively cost-free option that enables you to avoid causing harm to others. By declining to take this option, you arguably make it the case that a fair distribution of the risk of harm implies that you should suffer the harm of non-consensual tracking devices on your smartphone rather than risk others becoming infected with Covid-19. One argument in defence of this view appeals to the fact that most people would find it acceptable to demand that those who suspect they are infected with Covid-19 should self-isolate. Arguably, mandatory self-isolation is a greater intervention in daily life than downloading a tracking app (even if the latter lasts longer). Hence, if this demand is morally justified, then so too is the demand to download an app.

---

[12] We are assuming—justifiably so in the context of democracies, at least—that installing the infection tracking device, etc., has no serious harmful side effects for the innocent threat.

[13] Strictly speaking, they might not be able to consent, since they do not have a right against us that we do not surveil them. To accommodate this point, we could say that you can quasi-consent to an intervention against your body, mind, or property by communicating to others that you accept it, even if you do not have the right to refuse such an intervention.

[14] The same line of argument applies to omitting to self-isolate if the test is positive.

[15] This assumes, of course, that the tracking device is (reasonably believed by the person who refuses to download it to be) misused by the state to gain access other sorts of sensitive information about the app user. Perhaps this assumption is not satisfied in the case of some of less than fully democratic states in which the use of infection tracking apps is not fully consensual.

One interesting upshot of this is the following: superficially, by ticking the 'I agree' box on digital social media platforms and apps for mobile phones, we consent to sharing our personal information with a third party under conditions spelled out in the consent policies. However, privacy scholars have underlined that the consent policies are often very long and very difficult for laypersons to understand (Nissenbaum 2011). Also, the (social) price to users of opting out of such platforms is too high, which means that people are forced to accept the provider's terms. Hence, when ticking the 'I agree' box, we might not be sufficiently well informed, and the option of not consenting may not sufficiently acceptable for our consent to count as valid (Solove 2008; Tavani 2008).

By way of an example of Nissenbaum's concern, consider the Danish version of the Covid-19 tracking app. When you consent to the conditions of use, you consent to the health agencies keeping the information *as long as they consider it relevant*. Arguably, the fact that it is very hard to determine how long that will be, together with the use of impenetrable legalese, means that a tick in the 'I agree' box does not constitute valid consent (Adam Henschke and Patrick Taylor-Smith's chapters in this volume discuss some of these temporal issues with emergency pandemic surveillance).

A cynical response to this concern about the significant costs involve in knowing what one consents to is to say that the user can simply put greater effort into understanding the policies before accepting the terms of use—or alternatively, simply not use these apps and devices. However, one problem in this argument to the context of Covid-19 and the infection-tracking app is that the social cost of not downloading the app is not similar to that of opting out of social media platforms, where opting out typically involves significant costs, in the form of isolation from increasingly socially important fora etc.[16] Even so, other factors might render the option of not agreeing to the terms of use of Covid-19 tracking apps very costly. To return to our example two paragraphs ago, by appealing to social awareness, moral concern and respect for our fellow citizens ('*samfundssind*'), the Danish authorities have (so far) been very successful at promoting the use of the official Covid-19 tracking app.[17] Some worry, however, that in practice, the social shame associated with Covid-19-related irresponsible behaviour implies that people are subjected to a sufficient degree of coercion that their ticking the 'I agree' box does not to amount to valid consent.[18]

[16] See e.g., Solove's discussions on consent without a real choice (2008: 35).
[17] The Danish app has been downloaded 2.2 million times according to (Styrelsen for Patientsikkerhed 2021), which amounts to over one-third of the Danish population.
[18] Tech observers and scholars in Denmark have raised various worries concerning the Danish Covid-19 tracking app, e.g., Stine Bosse, who is Director of the Danish Tech Commission, Associate Professor at Copenhagen Business School Nanna Bonde Thylstrup, and Senior Researcher at The Danish Institute for Human Rights Rikke Frank Jørgensen (Jørgensen 2020).

If our argument is sound, then for some purposes at least, we can simply bypass such discussions about whether the sort of consent people give, when they tick 'I agree' boxes, amounts to valid consent. We can at least do so for the purpose of determining whether they are wronged, since, generally, their consent is not morally required in the first place. Again, this does not mean that this discussion might not be relevant for other purposes. Some might say, e.g., that current consent policies are manipulative, and that even manipulating people whose consent is not required can be wrongful in certain ways. However, such concerns are not those at play in most discussions of whether people's consent on social media, etc., is valid.

## Why Consent Might Matter Morally, Despite Liability

Suppose that our argument in the previous section is sound. If so, then consent is not morally required in relation to installing tracking apps on the smartphones of the many potential bearers of Covid-19 who negligently expose others to risk of infection. By negligently exposing others to the risk of death or serious harm, they have no right to refuse others taking certain relatively non-draconian defensive measures against them, such as installing Covid-19 tracking apps on their smartphone. This seems to run counter to the widespread assumption in many European countries that the use of such apps requires the consent of the user. Hence, in closing, we want to explain why our argument in the previous section does not imply that a consent-based approach to Covid-19-related tracking apps is not the morally preferable approach, even if other approaches not based on consent are morally permissible.

One set of concerns that might, in some cases at least, favour the voluntary use of tracking apps is purely pragmatic. If, for instance, it is not politically feasible to enforce a ban on *not* downloading the app, then it might be morally better to try to persuade people to download it voluntarily, even if we know that far from everyone will do so, rather than to seek to make it legally mandatory to use the app. Similarly, if we know that if they are forced to download tracking apps, many people will simply not turn on their smartphone (or, simply, turn off Bluetooth, in which case the tracking app does not function) in situations where they might transmit the disease, then making tracking apps legally mandatory will defeat the purpose.

These pragmatic concerns are important but perhaps less theoretically interesting.[19] Here, we are primarily interested in a different, non-pragmatic concern,

---

[19] The forced use of the apps in some countries such as China suggests that it is possible, if not politically favourable, to overcome these pragmatic difficulties. We thank a reviewer for pointing out the need to clarify this point.

related to the sort of disrespect that is argued to be inherent in paternalistic policies. Many believe that paternalistic policies are based on the supposition that people do not act in ways that promote their own good—or at least, not as much as the state does—and that basing policies on such a presupposition disrespects the citizens. Since the state ought not to treat its citizens with disrespect, it follows that the state ought not to treat it citizens paternalistically (Anderson 1999: 330; Quong 2011; Shiffrin 2000).[20]

However, imposing the non-consensual use of Covid-19 tracking apps on smartphone users is not a paternalistic policy. At least, it is not the case that when the state forces a particular citizen to download a tracking app, it does so for the good of that particular citizen. Rather, it does so first and foremost to benefit other citizens.[21] Hence, the state forces citizens to take action to help other citizens, because it foresees that forcing citizens to download the app better serves this end than leaving the decision up to the citizens themselves. This supposition is analogous to the supposition behind paternalistic policies that citizens will not make the right choices from the perspective of their own good. Here, however, the supposition is that citizens will not make the morally right choice. It seems undeniable that a supposition of this kind lies behind the drive to make the tracking app compulsory.[22] Our next claim is that if the state disrespects citizens when it does not trust them to promote their own good, then it also disrespects them when it does not trust them to make morally good choices, such as downloading a tracking app to reduce the risk to others of contracting Covid-19. In support of this conditional claim is the fact that we tend to be more offended when others criticize us for making immoral choices than when they criticize us for making imprudent ones.[23] Hence, if much liberal critique of paternalism is justified, then there is a reason to rely on consensual Covid-19 tracking apps, even if people are actually liable to having such apps imposed on them non-consensually.[24]

---

[20] For present purposes, we will leave open what the source of this moral injunction might be, e.g., whether treating citizens with concern and respect is a condition for the right to rule (Dworkin 2000) or whether it is a duty that the state owes to each citizen.

[21] We set aside the complication that, possibly, the state might be said to be engaging in collective paternalism, i.e., by forcing each citizen to act in a particular way it makes all citizens better off (reducing the risk of acquiring Covid-19).

[22] Some might deny this on the ground that the state might act out of a concern to avoid free riding, i.e., it supposes that the great majority of citizens will voluntarily use the app, but also that a tiny minority will free ride on others' moral choices.

[23] Some might object that this can hardly be disrespectful, since it is a fact that a lot of citizens will make immoral choices, and that the state does not disrespect anyone by supposing what is obviously true. Whether or not this is so, note that exactly the same line of argument applies to allegedly disrespectful policies, since it is a plain fact that all of us will often make imprudent choices.

[24] Note that similar concern about disrespect does not apply in paradigmatic cases of self-defence. For example, once I load my gun and point it in your direction, preparing to negligently see if it works by shooting, I can no longer complain that you disrespect me by assuming that I am about to make an immoral choice—I am in the process of doing so.

# Conclusion

All of us are threats to others, in the sense that we might transmit serious infection to them. Most of us are non-innocent threats, in that we are responsible for objectively unjust threats to other people's lives or health. Plausibly, infection tracking apps can help us fight epidemics, including the Covid-19 pandemic. Assuming that one does not live in an autocratic state in which there is a significant risk that the data that such apps generate will be misused for non-infection-related purposes, most of us are liable to have an infection-tracking app installed on our smartphones and to various relative moderate and appropriate interventions motivated by the information provided by those devices, e.g., compulsory testing and avoidance of risky behaviour. Accordingly, we are not wronged when this happens, and our consent is not required for such an intervention not to wrong us. Even so, there may be pragmatic as well as principled reasons why consensual surveillance schemes are morally preferable (e.g., in the absence of significant counterweighing moral costs, such as a much lower degree of use of the tracking app). In particular, we have argued, based on reasoning similar to that which grounds many liberals' view that paternalistic policies are disrespectful, that non-consensual surveillance schemes might be disrespectful, in that they send the message that citizens are likely to make immoral choices.

# References

Anderson, E. 1999. 'What Is the Point of Equality?' *Ethics* 109 (2): 287–337.

Bellaby, R. W. 2012. 'What's the Harm? The Ethics of Intelligence Collection'. *Intelligence and National Security* 27 (1): 93–117.

Clark, M. 2000. 'Self-Defence against the Innocent'. *Journal of Applied Philosophy* 17 (2): 145–55.

Diderichsen, A. and K. V. Rønn. 2017. 'Intelligence by Consent: On the Inadequacy of Just War Theory as a Framework for Intelligence Ethics'. *Intelligence and National Security* 32 (4): 479–93. https://doi.org/10.1080/02684527.2016.1270622

Dukakis, A. 2020. 'China rolls out software surveillance for the COVID-19 pandemic, alarming human rights advocates', *ABC NEWS*, 14 April 2020, available at: https://abcnews.go.com/International/china-rolls-software-surveillance-covid-19-pandemic-alarming/story [accessed 30 April 2023].

Dworkin, R. 2000. *Sovereign Virtue*. Cambridge, MA: Harvard University Press.

Jørgensen, R. F. 2020. 'DEBAT: Den danske smittestop-app har flyttet sig fra statslig overvågning til tech-giganter', *Danish Institute for Human Righs*, available at: https://menneskeret.dk/nyheder/debat-danske-smittestop-app-flyttet-statslig-over-vaagning-tech-giganter [accessed 30 April 2023].

Kleinig, J. 2009. 'The Ethical Perils of Knowledge Acquisition'. *Criminal Justice Ethics* 28 (2): 201–22. doi:10.1080/07311290903181218.

Lever, A. 2016. 'Democracy, Privacy and Security'. In *Privacy, Security and Accountability. Ethics, Law and Policy*, edited by Adam D. Moore, 105–24. London: Rowman & Littlefield.

Lippert-Rasmussen, K. 2020. 'Covid-19 "Tracing Apps", Quarantine, and Innocent Threats'. *Stockholm Centre for the Ethics of War and Peace*: http://stockholmcentre.org/covid-19-tracing-apps-quarantine-and-innocent-threats/

Lyon, D. 2014. 'Surveillance, Snowden, and Big Data: Capacities, Consequences, Critique'. *Big Data & Society*. doi: https://doi.org/10.1177/2053951714541861

Macnish, K. 2014. 'Just Surveillance? Towards a Normative Theory of Surveillance'. *Surveillance & Society* 12 (1): 142–53.

Macnish, K. 2015. 'An Eye for an Eye: Proportionality and Surveillance'. *Ethical Theory and Moral Practice* 18: 529–48.

Macnish, K. 2018. 'Government Surveillance and Why Defining Privacy Matters in a Post-Snowden World'. *Journal of Applied Philosophy* 35 (2): doi: 10.1111/japp.12219

Marx, G. T. 1998. 'Ethics for the New Surveillance'. *The Information Society* 14 (3): 171–85.

McMahan, J. 1994. 'Self-defense and the problem of the innocent attacker'. *Ethics* 104 (2): 252–90.

McMahan, J. 2009. *Killing in Wars*. Oxford: Oxford University Press.

Nathan, C. 2017. 'Liability to Deception and Manipulation: The Ethics of Undercover Policing'. *Journal of Applied Philosophy* 34 (3): 370–88.

Nissenbaum, H. 2011. 'A Contextual Approach to Privacy Online'. *Daedalus* 140 (4): 32–48.

Nozick, R. 1974. *Anarchy, State, and Utopia*. Oxford: Basil Blackwell.

Quong, J. 2011. *Liberalism without Perfection*. Oxford: Oxford University Press.

Quong, J. 2020. *The Morality of Defensive Force*. Oxford: Oxford University Press.

Rønn, K. V. and K. Lippert-Rasmussen. 2020. 'Out of Proportion? On Surveillance and the Proportionality Requirement'. *Ethical Theory and Moral Practice* 23 (1): 181–99.

Shiffrin, S. 2000. 'Paternalism, Unconscionability Doctrine, and Accommodation'. *Philosophy & Public Affairs* 29: 205–50.

Solove, D. J. 2008. *Understanding Privacy*. Cambridge, MA: Harvard University Press.

Stahl, T. 2016. 'Indiscriminate Mass Surveillance and the Public Sphere'. *Ethics and Information Technology* 18 (1): 33–9.

Stanley, J. and S. G. Granick. 'The Limits of Location Tracking in an Epidemic'. *AUCL* (8 April), available at: https://www.aclu.org/sites/default/files/field_document/limits_of_location_tracking_in_an_epidemic.pdf [accessed 30 April 2023].

Stoddart, E. 2014. 'Challenging "Just Surveillance Theory": A Response to Kevin Macnish's "Just Surveillance? Towards a Normative Theory of Surveillance"'. *Surveillance Society* 12: 158–63.

Styrelsen for Patientsikkerhed. 2021. "Smitte|stop." 2021. https://smittestop.dk [accessed 8 April 2021].

Tavani, H. T. 2008. 'Informational Privacy: Concepts, Theories, and Controversies'. In *The Handbook of Information and Computer Ethics*, edited by K. E. Himma and H. T. Tavani, 131–64. Hoboken, New Jersey: John Wiley & Sons, Incorporated.

Thomson, J. J. 1991. 'Self-Defense'. *Philosophy and Public Affairs* 20 (1): 53–66.

Uniacke, S. 2011. 'Proportionality and Self-Defense'. *Law and Philosophy* 30 (3): 253–72.

Vaughan, A. 2020. 'There are many reasons why covid-19 contact-tracing apps may not work', *New Scientist*, 17 April, available at: https://www.newscientist.com/article/2241041-there-are-many-reasons-why-covid-19-contact-tracing-apps-may-not-work/ [accessed 30 April 2023].

WHO 2020. 'Ethical considerations to guide the use of digital proximity tracking technologies for COVID-19 contact tracing' 28 May 2020, *World Health Organization*, available at: https://www.who.int/publications/i/item/WHO-2019-nCoV-Ethics_Contact_tracing_apps-2020.1 [accessed 30 April 2023].

# 7

# Digital Contact Tracing Applications (DCTAs)

## Public Health Ethics and Emergency Surveillance

*Sahar Latheef*

## Introduction

Infectious disease surveillance involves investigating how an infectious disease spreads within a community (Murray and Cohen 2017: 222–9). Contact tracing is one of the methods undertaken by public health officials to identify, assess and manage people who have been exposed to a disease. Effective contact tracing contributes to preventing transmission of disease within the community (Thomas Craig et al. 2021). The SARS-CoV-2 pandemic (from here on Covid-19) has seen an increase in uptake of Digital Contact Tracing Applications (DCTAs),[1] and with this an interest in ethical issues such as individual liberty, privacy, and agency (Cattuto and Spina 2020: 228–35). To assuage concerns regarding the impact on individual privacy, technology companies such as Google and Apple have stated that the data collected and stored would be anonymous or de-identified in some form (Bradford et al. 2020). However, for contact tracing to be useful the data would need to identify individuals to some degree in order to trace, notify contacts and investigate outbreaks.

At its core, the problem that this chapter is concerned with is this—DCTAs can collect large amounts of personally identifiable information. The approach taken by public health officials in using DCTAs could impact individual rights such as autonomy and the right to informed consent. Approaches that lean towards mandatory use of DCTAs could impact autonomy and informed consent more than other approaches. Therefore, careful considerations ought to be made in identifying morally justified trade-offs. When can we balance individual rights against protection of public health? In this chapter, I look at how DCTAs have been used and how this impacts autonomy and informed consent. I propose that

---

[1] I use the abbreviation DCTA to refer to all forms digital contact tracing applications and digital health products. Other similar terms used in literature are Digital Contact Tracing Technology (DCTT), DCT Systems, Contact Tracing Applications (CTAs).

Sahar Latheef, *Digital Contact Tracing Applications (DCTAs): Public Health Ethics and Emergency Surveillance* In: *The Ethics of Surveillance in Times of Emergency*. Edited by: Kevin Macnish and Adam Henschke, Oxford University Press.

in specific public health emergencies such as the Covid-19 pandemic, mandatory use of DCTAs could be morally justified in order to prioritize public health over individual rights given that it meets certain justificatory conditions (discussed later in this chapter).

Given those points and to support my proposition, I will assess attempts at achieving a balance between two (seemingly) incompatible aspects; individual rights and the greater good of public health and analyse claims arguing in favour of one over the other. My analysis will be based on two theoretical approaches: (1) what I will call a bioethics approach which places informed consent among the core values and a justification on infringing a core value is challenging at best; and (2) what I will call a public health ethics approach, that places comparatively less significance on individual rights such as informed consent and a higher value on public health as a public good warranting collective action. In my analysis, I aim to demonstrate that given the state of emergency and extreme circumstances[2] during a pandemic the scale of Covid-19, we ought to follow a public health ethics approach even if it impacts individual autonomy and informed consent to some extent, until such time when the risks are not as high, and more information is available.

The first part of this chapter looks at DCTA technology and how it is used as an epidemiological tool. I will focus on the technology's features such as proximity detection and data collection, storage and sharing. Following this, I look at how DCTAs are used focusing on three types of approach: a maximum, middle, and minimum approach. I demonstrate that a combination of the features of DCTAs and how they are used impacts autonomy and informed consent, and therefore contributes to the discussions presented later in this chapter where I examine if mandatory use of DCTAs could be morally justified.

The second part looks at why we need DCTAs. In this part, I highlight the advantages that DCTAs offer, both potential and actual. I look at how DCTAs could contribute to early detection in diseases with high rates of transmission, morbidity, and mortality, when significant proportion of individuals are asymptomatic or pre-symptomatic, and indirectly contribute to reducing lockdowns and burden on healthcare systems.

The final part provides an analysis on informed consent and autonomy based on two approaches: (1) what I call a bioethics approach and (2) what I call a public health ethics approach. Taking a bioethics approach, I examine whether the use of DCTAs and infringements on autonomy and informed consent could be morally justified. Following on, I compare this to a public health ethics approach where I look at three conditions; necessity, effectiveness and least infringement to examine moral justification using DCTAs. I also propose two other justifications:

---

[2] I use the term extreme circumstances here to refer to the high levels of risk and uncertainty during the Covid-19 pandemic.

fairness in distributing burdens and protecting vulnerable groups in the population as possible justifications in this context.

## DCTAs: A Look at How the Technology Works and Approach Taken to Implement Their Use

### How DCTAs Work

There are various types of DCTAs. How DCTAs function depends on the technology design. The different types of DCTAs vary in the extent to which they
impact an individual's privacy, i.e., ranging from very intrusive DCTAs that collect
large amounts of personally identifiable information to less intrusive DCTAs that
collect minimal information. The basic architecture of DCTAs consists of a mobile
device, e.g., smartphone and a software application installed on the device
designed to collect information (data). In the following paragraphs, I will look at
the key features, such as proximity detection, data collection, data storage, and
data sharing These features have (potential) ethical implications, as they determine the extent to which DCTAs allow informed consent and autonomy (Jacob
and Lawarée 2021: 44–58).

Proximity detection is the feature that allows DCTAs to keep a record of an
individual's movements while in the community. There are two main ways
DCTAs could carry out proximity detection. For example, via Bluetooth Low
Energy (BLE) signals and GPS triangulation. BLE-based DCTAs communicate
with nearby smartphones and make records of other DCTAs within a specified
distance for a specific period of time. When a person receives a notification of a
positive test result, the location data is decrypted and made accessible to public
health officials. The phone numbers of other individuals that the positive person
has come into contact are obtained by health officials. The purpose here is to then
notify the contacts of the individual who could be potentially infected, so that they
may get tested and quarantine or isolate. Proximity detection can also be achieved
via GPS triangulation with nearby mobile phone communication towers (Miller
and Smith 2021: 366–71). GPS based DCTAs record detailed information on an
individuals' whereabouts, e.g., location addresses, date, time, and duration. As
GPS based DCTAs are designed to collect and handle more data than BLEs, and
often uses personally identifiable information in conjunction with location details,
they can provide a more comprehensive picture than that provided by BLEs.
Based on this information, we can see that there is a range in/degrees of level of
intrusion on individual privacy depending on the type of proximity detection
method (Miller and Smith 2021).

To minimize the impact on individual privacy, the data collected can be
anonymized to some extent allowing some degree of protection of individual

privacy.³ Anonymization is when data collected does not include information that could easily identify an individual. Instead, it provides details of locations of where an individual was during the infectious period. Non-anonymized data consists of more detailed information such as location specifications and medical information such as details of symptoms and test dates. The level of infringement on individual privacy has been an important factor in assessing ethical issues relating to the use of DCTAs. As mentioned earlier, for contact tracing to be useful, the data would need to identify individuals to some degree in order to trace, notify contacts, and investigate outbreaks. I will return to this point later in the chapter when discussing efficacy as a necessary condition in the justification of mandatory use of DCTAs. That is, if the technology is not effective in achieving the intended outcome, we may not be able to morally justify their mandatory use.

The level of intrusion on individual privacy could also depend on data storage methods. There are three types of data storage mechanisms; a centralized mechanism using a centralized server, a partially centralized mechanism storing selective data only from some individuals (i.e., individuals who have tested positive for the disease), or a decentralized storage mechanism where data is stored on individual phones (Kahn 2020). Centralized storage allows technology companies that develop or host DCTAs to access data as well as public health officials, therefore more intrusive to individual privacy (Lodders and Paterson 2020: 154). However, centralized storage also allows multiple health agencies easier access to data resulting in easier/more efficient contact tracing processes. However, this also makes it easier for governmental agencies such as law enforcement easy access to the data even if it is not related to a public health response (Greenleaf and Kemp 2021). This relatively easy access to data for reasons that are not related to public health emergencies has contributed to the concerns regarding privacy and data protection.

To address privacy concerns, some DCTAs use decentralized data collection and storage methods. For example, consider the 'COVIDSafe' DCTA used in Australia (Miller and Smith 2021). Decentralized mechanisms make it more challenging to access the data (hence privacy preserving). Whilst this method is considered privacy preserving, the longer lag times to access data has a flow on effect causing delays in the contact tracing process. The delays are more significant in multi-agency responses when more than one agency requires access to the decentralized data. Each individual agency would then need to request access to the data stored on individual phones rather than a centralized mechanism where all data is available in the one place. The point here is that, whilst some forms of data storage allow for greater preservation of individual privacy, it comes at a cost

---

³ I recognize here that even with anonymized data, there may still be privacy concerns arising from the aggregation and analysis of non-personal information. See Henschke (2017) for more on this.

in the form of decreased efficiency in contact tracing, the very reason the data was needed in the first instance (White and Van Basshuysen 2021a: 23, 2021b).[4]

In addition to the impact on individual privacy, proximity detection and data-sharing functionalities create blurred boundaries in regard to obtaining informed consent. Proximity detection features gather information on a primary individual, and on secondary individuals with respect to the primary individual. For example, if I am identified as at risk of being infectious, when I give consent for the health agencies to access my data, I am giving access to information not just about myself but also giving information about myself and other individuals who I have come into contact with within the certain timeframe and in a specific location. Later in this chapter, I will look at the complexities arising from consenting in this nature and what this means in respect to the moral justifications in mandatory use of DCTAs.

## Approaches Taken in Using DCTAs

John Hopkins *Project on Ethics and Governance of Digital Contact Tracing Technologies* placed DCTAs into three broad categories based on how they function and how they are used as an epidemiological tool. These categories are a maximal, middle, and a minimal approach (Kahn 2020). A maximal approach consists of DCTAs most intrusive to individual privacy, where a broad range of data is collected such as location specific data and medical information. This data is not anonymized and provides a clear picture of an individual's whereabouts and other personal details. DCTAs store data on a centralized server where is it made available to multiple agencies as needed. In some countries such as South Korea, the data collected from DCTAs are integrated with data from other sources such as credit card companies, public transport information, facial recognition cameras, and social media (Ryan 2020). Often, though not always, a maximal approach involves mandatory use of DCTAs making this approach one that impacts autonomy and informed consent the most.

The more commonly used DCTAs are those that fall in the middle ground. The middle ground approach consists of two subtypes: (1) collection of deidentified data automatically stored on a central database; or (2) collection of personal identification data stored via decentralized mechanisms such on individual phones, rather than centrally. In the latter, the data is stored on user's phones for a specific period of time. Some middle ground approaches allow individuals who have received positive test results to voluntarily upload their data to a specific

---

[4] I recognize here that even with anonymized data, there may still be privacy concerns arising from the aggregation and analysis of non-personal information. For more on this see Henschke (2017: 1–334).

website accessible by health officials. Health officials can then analyse the data to identify Covid-19 positive individuals, locations, and times of exposure, and broadcast a redacted version of this data to other relevant users. Variations in functionality occur across the range of middle-ground DCTAs. They key element common to DCTAs falling into this category is that there is some form of privacy preservation in either using deidentified data, or involving a voluntary choice from individuals in sharing/disclosing identifiable data with public health officials, allowing some degree of autonomy and consent.

A minimal approach is where data collection is via decentralized Privacy Preserving Proximity Tracking (PPPT) methods (e.g., developed by Google and Apple) (White and Van Basshuysen 2021a). Minimal approaches use BLE signals that record contacts between mobile phone users within a specific distance during a specific time. Other details such as location and personal identification information are not collected. When an individual receives a positive test result, other individuals that have come into contact with the now infectious individual can be notified either automatically, or at the discretion of the individual, depending on the technology design. Individuals receives a notification alerting them to a possible exposure with a timestamp to indicate when the exposure has occurred, but no other data is shared. Often, though not always, using these types of DCTAs are encouraged and not mandated.

## In Support of DCTAs

Considering how DCTAs work and the potential impact on autonomy and informed consent, do we need DCTAs at all? The Covid-19 pandemic saw a significant global uptake of DCTAs. By December 2020, approximately seventy-four countries were using DCTAs in their response to the pandemic (Storeng and De Bengy Puyvallée 2021). However, this is not the first time that DCTAs have been used to in responding to infectious disease outbreaks. For example, in the management of diseases such as Ebola (Danquah et al. 2019: 810), Middle East Respiratory Syndrome (MERS), HIV, Chlamydia and Gonorrhoea (Kahn 2020). DCTAs were used to facilitate case interviews, send partner notifications for Sexually Transmitted Infections (STIs), and as a form of digital record keeping, rather than a means of digitizing or automating the contact tracing process. That said, the Covid-19 pandemic saw an unprecedented rise in the use of DCTAs. Given the likelihood of ongoing pandemics and increased antibiotic resistance, we are likely to face increased challenges from infectious diseases, and so DCTAs are going to be persistent technologies into the future.

Given that DCTAs can potentially infringe or violate people's privacy, we need to ask the questions; how do DCTAs contribute to response against infectious disease outbreaks? And is this better than what manual contact tracing can offer?

DCTAs have the potential to provide faster data collection, and can handle large volumes of data concurrently, than manual contact tracing. This is required in situations where early detection, communication and intervention is crucial. The following paragraphs will discuss these factors in support of DCTAs.

## Early Detection

DCTAs provide the means for public health officials to carry out early detection of infected individuals. Early detection is crucial in outbreaks where a disease has a high rate of transmission, infects a large number of people in the population, significant proportion of infections cause people to become seriously ill or result in deaths (high percentages of morbidity and mortality), and have higher percentages of asymptomatic and pre-symptomatic individuals. These are just some of the factors that drove public health reliance on DCTAs during the Covid-19 pandemic. According to the World Health Organization, as of 20 February 2022 there were over 422 million confirmed cases and approximately 5.8 million deaths globally (World Health Organization 2022). In addition to lives lost, large numbers of people will suffer from symptoms, some serious enough to warrant hospitalization and intensive care. Early detection contributes to early intervention, increasing the likelihood of individuals receiving the necessary medical attention including life-saving intervention, thereby, reducing mortality rates. Early intervention also reduces the likelihood of individuals experiencing long term side effects after recovery. A study published in Nature 2021, investigated the impact of DCTAs providing one of the first sets of empirical evidence in support of DCTAs as an epidemiological tool. This study investigated the National Health Service (NHS) Covid-19 app usage in England and Wales between September 2020 and December 2020 and demonstrated that for each individual notified, one case of Covid-19 was averted. During this period, approximately 16.5 million people used the NHS app and the app had sent approximately 1.7 million exposure notifications. This study, based on both modelling and statistical methodologies, demonstrated the number of cases averted during this period was approximately 284, 000 based on modelling and 594, 000 based on statistics (Wymant et al. 2021).

DCTAs provide an advantage over manual contact tracing methods in response to situations where there is a high percentage of asymptomatic and pre-symptomatic individuals. In Covid-19 epidemiology, asymptomatic individuals make up approximately 17–20 per cent of the infected population (Pollock and Lancaster 2020), and 50 per cent of the transmission occur early in the infection period prior to symptom development (Parker et al. 2020). Epidemiologists indicate that infectious period lasts seven to thirteen days and in some cases virus shedding was detected twenty days after infection (Chowdhury and Oommen 2020). A significant proportion of transmission (some as high as 50 per cent) occurs between asymptomatic individuals (Johansson et al. 2021), and transmissibility could extend for approximately three days before onset of symptoms for symptomatic individuals (i.e., pre-symptomatic transmission). Large numbers of asymptomatic and pre-symptomatic individuals make early detection challenging for manual contact tracing as it is more likely that individuals are not aware that they are infectious or the infectious period commences before tests results can be produced or acted upon (Park et al. 2020: 967). Considering the likelihood of being asymptomatic or pre-symptomatic, an individual could be unknowingly infectious in the community for days or even weeks, potentially exposing a large number of people to the disease. Studies show that in some extreme cases one infected individual could in turn infect up to thirty-two individuals (Maccari and Cagno 2021). In such situations, manual contact tracing efforts alone may not be sufficient to capture all the contacts of an infectious individual. Some individuals could also find it challenging to recall all of the locations that they have visited or details of all of the other people that they may have come in to contact. Relying on manual contact tracing alone also means relying on individuals to recall all of this information. DCTAs having the capacity to record an individual's whereabouts in real-time could offer a reliable alternative in providing a more accurate picture of an individual's whereabouts.

## DCTAs Indirectly Contribute to Reducing Lockdowns and Burden on Healthcare System

By providing a means to reduce transmission during an outbreak with high infection rates, DCTAs indirectly contribute to reducing the likelihood of measures such as the number of lockdowns or the duration of lockdowns a city or state could undergo. Lockdowns as a public health measure provides a means to socially distance and prevent people from gathering in areas where there is a risk of transmission, and are particularly important if there are limited treatments or prevention measures like vaccines available. In the Covid-19 pandemic, some countries such as Australia implemented significant lockdowns at a national level, that applied to everyone whether they were at immediate risk, affected, or vaccinated against the virus (Miller and Smith 2021).

In an examination of the public health measures during the Covid-19 pandemic, Parker and colleagues suggest that lockdowns are justified as a public health measure, when there is insufficient, accurate or reliable information regarding the risks status of individuals or specific locations (Parker et al. 2020). By providing information regarding risk status of individuals and details of locations where transmission occurs, DCTAs allow public health officials to implement more specific measures instead of blanket lockdowns in larger areas. Parker et al. state:

> The justification of blanket lockdowns would be weaker were it possible to manage physical distancing in a more evidence-based, risk-adjusted way. Were this so, it would remain the case that limiting the movements of those people who presented a high risk would be justified. It would not, however, be justified to restrict the movements of those individuals (and possibly populations) who were reliably known not to be contributing to this risk. Rapid contact tracing enabled by the mobile phone app described above—combined with accurate testing—has the potential to be a tool of this kind. The evidence suggests the app has the potential to enable some (likely many) people to return more quickly to their lives. This evidence puts pressure on justifications for blanket lockdowns.   (Parker et al. 2020)

The point here is that, while DCTAs might be privacy invasive and impact individual rights, the impact is comparatively less than measures such as blanket lockdowns infringing on basic rights and liberties for a greater number of people.

In the above paragraphs, I have put forward a case in support of DCTAs focusing on the advantages they offer over manual contact tracing methods. This defence is not without caveats. There are some functional differences between manual contact tracing and DCTAs that currently prevents DCTAS being used as a sole contact tracing method. Manual contact tracing has been used for decades in response to infectious diseases. Over this time, the manual contact tracing process has been trialled and tested, whereas DCTAs have only recently been implemented on a large scale similar to the Covid-19 pandemic. Importantly, trialling DCTAs at this scale is relatively new, so there are limits to what we can learn and extrapolate from the Covid-19 examples. As with any new technology, it is reasonable to expect limitations that were not foreseen ahead of implementation. For example, manual contact tracers interact with individuals who are either confirmed cases or suspected cases and not with the broader general public. This human-to-human interaction provides opportunities to clarify and eliminate misconceptions and errors in gathering the relevant information. DCTAs do not yet have a robust mechanism to verify false positive errors. Until the limitations can be addressed, DCTAs may be an effective measure in supporting manual contact tracing efforts and not replace manual methods altogether as the primary means of contact tracing. I discuss the importance of efficacy in the next section of this chapter, where I examine when mandatory use of DCTAs can be morally justified.

## DCTAs, Autonomy, and Informed Consent

Can we justify the use of DCTAs even if they infringe autonomy and informed consent? In this section, I will examine the answer to this question based on two approaches: (1) what I will call a bioethics approach which places autonomy and informed consent among the core values and any infringement of a core value may not be justified; and (2) what I will call a public health ethics approach where public health is considered a public good and requires collective action. This approach prioritizes health of the population over individual rights. I will demonstrate that in response to a pandemic the scale of Covid-19, could be morally justified. As such, we ought to take a public health approach where mandatory use of DCTAs, even if it impacts autonomy and informed consent.

## A Bioethics Approach

Informed consent, a concept that has its origins in medicine and biomedical research, is one of the core concepts of bioethics. Beauchamp and Childress conceptualize informed consent in two ways: (1) informed consent as an individual's autonomous authorization; and (2) as a social practice in an institutional context which forms the legal or institutionally effective form of informed consent (Beauchamp 2011). The first meaning of informed consent is a means of ensuring the individual gives consent only if the individual has substantial understanding of what they are consenting to and is free from control by external forces. Informed consent is an autonomous and intentional authorization by an individual or a self-determining choice.

The second aspect of informed consent is as a social practice, whereby informed consent applies to a legally or institutionally effective approval given by an individual (Beauchamp and Childress 2009). Here, informed consent is a mechanism to legally protect the individual giving consent and the institution or authority receiving consent. Less emphasis is placed on autonomous authorization or self-determination; rather, the focus is on legal liability or liability for injury. This aspect of informed consent is determined by laws and rules that govern the process of obtaining consent. In the case where an individual may claim compensation for injury, damages, or harm, it will be examined if the legally acceptable form of informed consent was obtained. If consent was obtained, it could be deemed as the individual has knowingly accepted the risks of the decision and has discharged responsibility of the authority/institution as being responsible for the risk-related outcomes. According to Beauchamp and Childress, it is possible for an individual to give informed consent in the first sense but without giving consent in the second sense (Beauchamp and Childress 2009). A decision could be autonomous and intentional but not be a legally acceptable form of informed consent. It is also possible for an individual to give consent that is legally acceptable but may not be autonomous and intentional.

Consider the mandatory use of DCTAs as discussed above. Some mandatory approaches involve punitive measures such as fines, and in some extreme situations, imprisonment for non-compliance. Mandatory use of centralized DCTAs under a maximal approach, as described in the first section of this chapter, is a prima facie case of circumventing informed consent and autonomy. In some countries such as South Korea and Israel, mandatory use of DCTAs were implemented in conjunction with additional surveillance measures.[5] Taking a bioethics approach, it would be challenging to provide a moral justification for the mandatory use of DCTAs in this manner as it overrides an individual's right to make an informed and autonomous decision.

Next, consider mandatory implementation of decentralized DCTAs. Decentralized DCTAs allow some level of user discretion in sharing data. When an individual consents to use DCTAs and share their data, it could be considered a legally acceptable form of consenting but may not be morally justified. The reason for this is that, by mandating use of DCTAs, it impacts informed consent and autonomy even if the technology design may allow individuals to choose whether or not to share their data. For example, when using decentralized DCTAs, I am able to choose whether or not to share my data with public health agencies, as the data is not automatically uploaded to a central server, but under mandatory public health policies I am still required to share my data if I have visited a high-risk location. This gives me some capacity to choose in one instance, but takes away my ability to choose/consent in another. Is this an autonomous decision that I make? I propose that I have not made an autonomous decision as one aspect of the decision (i.e., in choosing whether or not to use DCTAs) did not allow for an informed consent.

Consider the voluntary implementation of decentralized DCTAs as discussed in the middle and minimal approaches. Decentralized DCTAs allows some form of choice[6] by offering individuals the discretion on whether or not to share their data. The voluntariness aspect in the middle to minimal approaches also allow for some degree of autonomy. If individuals can choose whether or not to use DCTAs, it could perhaps be morally justified under a bioethics approach. However, if this voluntary use of DCTAs is a condition to other factors such as in determining whether an individual can move freely within the community and access services required for their day to day lives, then this decision only allows for *some* degree of autonomy (or perhaps none depending on the type of conditions). For example, in

---

[5] Additional surveillance measures such as mobile phone companies, mandatory facial recognition, and social media (Ryan 2020).

[6] Variations in technology design allows for different types of informed consent, such as broad consent, meta consent, specific consent, and dynamic consent. The various types of informed consent, each with their respective ethical implications are discussed elsewhere in the literature. See Steinsbekk et al. (2013) and Budin-Ljøsne et al. (2017).

Australia, at the beginning of the pandemic in 2020, public health responses included disincentives to influence people in using DCTAs. With the rise in community transmissions and as states went into cycles of lockdown and varying degrees of isolation, the governments pushed to increase DCTA usage by linking the percentage of DCTAs downloaded to the possibility of having fewer lock-downs and isolations requirements (Goggin 2020). In situations such as this, the autonomy preserving component of informed consent does not lie solely on the first order decision (choosing to use DCTAs or not); but also on the second-order decision (choosing to face fines and other restrictions). In short, being compelled to give consent to something is not fully informed consent. On a bioethics view, which places significant weight on informed consent, such middle approaches might not be justifiable.

Voluntary use of DCTAs that fall in the middle to minimal approach, pose another complication with respect to their proximity detection features. The way proximity detection in decentralized DCTAs work is it involves leveraging informed consent obtained from one individual as the basis to obtain information about another. For example, I have consented to the use of DCTAs and to keep a record of my whereabouts on my phone. The DCTA has been recording my whereabouts for days and weeks. Weeks into using a DCTA, I have now started developing symptoms. Public health officials access the data on my phone, as I have consented to this, and notify the people with whom I have come into contact within the period of time I was deemed to be infectious in the community. In this case, I have now consented not just for myself (health officials to access information about my whereabouts) but also for my friends and family whom which public health officials now have information about them attending specific locations. This would not be ethically contentious if my friends and family have separately consented to the use of DCTAs and information about their where-abouts to be made accessible to health officials. However, if among this group of individuals, there was a person who has not consented to her whereabouts being made known, I have by consenting to myself, also consented for her without her consenting for herself, and infringed on her right to privacy. DCTAs that fall in the spectrum of middle to minimal approach, depending on technology design, have the potential to infringe informed consent and autonomy.

A counter argument to the above point is, given how DCTAs work, each individual would need to have the DCTA downloaded on their phone for them to be identified as a contact. As such, all individuals would have consented to the use of DCTAs. Therefore, when I consent to myself and for others, it would not make a difference as others have individually consented to the use of DCTAs. The question here is then, does the sum of all individual consents equal to one broad/collective consent for all? I would argue that even if one of my friends have consented to use DCTAs, she may not necessarily consent to share details of her whereabouts in relation to me or another specific individual. Taking a strong bioethics view to this, voluntary use of DCTAs, even if decentralized in design, may not be morally justified due to how proximity detection works, because of how it infringes on informed consent and autonomy.

Does the requirement of informed consent carry more moral weight in some situations and not the others? Discussions in the literature suggest that the need for informed consent is dependent on context. This is similar to the concept of varying levels of voluntariness and degrees of autonomy provided in bioethics literature (Beauchamp and Childress 2013). For example, in a research context, obtaining informed consent is more important when research is conducted on vulnerable populations and dependent how intrusive the research is on individual rights (Beauchamp 2011). Similarly, in a medical setting, the requirement of obtaining a voluntary informed consent is more important when dealing with invasive treatments, than compared to the routine non-invasive treatments. The importance of informed consent has some form of contextual dependence on the degree of harm on the individual (Eyal 2019; Beauchamp 2011). Following this scalar approach to informed consent, the Nuffield Council on Bioethics proposed an intervention ladder showing that the more invasive measures ought to provide a greater justification than the lesser invasive measures (Nuffield Council on Bioethics 2007). A similar approach to this is evident in the public health ethics domain when discussing the need for informed consent based on the purpose to which is it is being sought. In the following section, I will look at how informed consent and autonomy is discussed under a public health ethics approach and look at situations where mandatory use of DCTAS could be morally justified.

## A Public Health Ethics Approach

In contrast to the bioethics approach, the primary concern of public health ethics is the health of the entire population. In this sense it is non-individualistic (Childress et al. 2002). According to ethicists such as Onora O'Neill, public health is a public good and can only be realized at a collective level. O'Neill states that the provision of public goods cannot be dependent on individualized rights such as informed consent and must be made compulsory (O'Neill 2004: 1133–6). For example, road, food, water, and pharmaceutical safety measures. Following Seumas Miller, like these, public health is a collective good as collective goods are 'jointly produced goods that ought to be produced and made available to the whole community [and] since they are desirable goods and ones to which the members of the community have joint moral rights' (Miller 2014).

In defence of mandatory public health measures, O'Neill calls to set aside debates about informed consent and instead advocates for the consideration of permissible limits of mandatory use of public health goods. O'Neill buttresses her argument on John Stuart Mill's harms principle, which proposes that compulsory state interventions can only be justified under the narrow scope of preventing harm to others (O'Neill 2004). Discussions in favour of public health often view public health measures as a form of preventing harm to others and are therefore justified in taking precedence over individual liberty, and in extension right to informed consent and autonomy (O'Neill 2004; Nuffield Council on Bioethics 2007; Powers et al. 2012). In considering public health measures such as preventing transmission of infectious disease, the link to 'preventing harm to others' is more direct and straightforward than compared to other public health measures. Following this reasoning, one could also propose that public health measures such as the use of DCTAs could be justified given that they play a role in reducing the harm to others, even at the cost of individual rights.

A slightly different view to O'Neill's on mandatory public health ethics is one that is provided by Powers and Faden, stating that there is a plurality of justifications for liberty limiting public health policies other than preventing harm to others. Powers and Faden propose that not all liberties carry equal moral weight, and liberties that are in need of the greatest protection are those that are important to the value of self-determination (Powers and Faden 2013: 45–9). Even then, such liberties can be defeated by a plurality of reasons. The main liberties that merit protection against state interference of individual choice are those that link individual choice/self-determination to well-being.

The point I make here is that public health ethicists, whilst calling for less emphasis on individual's right to choose, do not disagree with the bioethics view on the value placed on an individual's right to informed consent. On the public health ethics view, individual autonomy and a right to self-determination is acknowledged as necessary to well-being. Instead, what proponents of the public health framework such as Powers and Faden suggest, is that not all regulatory measures or public health policies require the *same* level of justification. I extend this argument in defence of mandatory public health measures such as use of DCTAs (proven they meet certain conditions as discussed in the following paragraphs).

Childress et al. (2002) provide a different perspective on public health ethics by offering what they refer to as general moral considerations[7] as a defence for the pursuit of public health. Different to the approach by O'Neill, this view acknowledges that the general moral considerations are not absolute and could sometimes be in conflict with each other and each may have to yield in some situations. For example, when respect for autonomy is in conflict with the need for collective

---

[7] General moral considerations offered here as a means to avoid commitment to a particular theory or methods. Rather as means that is compatible with several approaches. The authors look at the moral appeals made by public health agents in discussing and justifying their actions and debates about moral issues. Their general moral considerations include; producing benefits, preventing harms, producing maximal benefit, distributing benefits and burdens, ensuring public participation, respecting autonomy, protecting privacy, keeping promises and commitments, transparency, and building and maintaining trust.

action. In such situations, it would be necessary to establish a mechanism to prioritize which general moral consideration ought to take priority. Childress et al., offer five justificatory conditions to determine which general moral consideration ought to take priority should it conflict with another. These justificatory conditions are: necessity, least infringement, effectiveness, proportionality, and public justification (Allen and Selgelid 2017).

These conditions can be used to determine if and when the use of DCTAs prioritizing public health over individual rights such as autonomy and informed consent could be justified. Considering how DCTAs are being used, and assuming a public health emergency similar to Covid-19, I will focus on the first three conditions: necessity, effectiveness, and least infringement, as they are more relevant to this discussion. These three conditions are to some extent interdependent on each other (as discussed below). Proportionality,[8] whilst relevant, will be excluded from my analysis, as it is discussed in detail elsewhere in the literature.[9]

Public health interventions ought to be necessary in achieving the intended goal. Where there are multiple options available, the necessity condition requires that the cost of intervention is one that cannot be avoided in seeking the end goal (Allen and Selgelid 2017). Childress et al. (2002) state that 'the fact that a policy will infringe a general moral consideration provides a strong moral reason to seek an alternative strategy that is less morally troubling.' The particular intervention must be unavoidable. On this, the burden of proof lies on those that propose mandatory measures, that they must provide evidence that the mandatory measures are necessary.

In the case of DCTAs, if their use infringes a general moral consideration such as informed consent and autonomy, the necessity condition requires that proof of necessity be provided and that this is a measure that cannot be avoided. As discussed earlier in this chapter, research investigating DCTAs used in England and Wales, has demonstrated that, for every individual consenting to notification, one case of Covid-19 was averted, thereby averting approximately 284,000 to 594,000 cases (Wymant et al. 2021). This research, and others similar to it, could be a starting point in demonstrating that DCTAs are a necessary epidemiological tool in response to a pandemic such as Covid-19. Further research with similar aims, are needed to strengthen this justification.

If the general moral conditions also requires that choice of intervention must be the least costly, how do we measure this? A commonly accepted guideline on how

---

[8] Proportionality, referring to the measure implemented being proportional to what it aims to achieve.

[9] I note that there is some overlap between the conditions of least infringement and proportionality. Least infringement involves comparing options to determine which one is least costly. This is similar to proportionality in that it compares the different outcomes and assess these outcomes based on their impact or cost to determine which one is less costly. There are several methods of calculating proportionality which I will not go into detail here. In this chapter I will use least infringement condition as it used to determine how choosing one moral condition impacts another instead of a cost–benefit analysis of using DCTAs in general. For more on proportionality calculations see Henschke (2018).

to choose between alternative conditions do not exist, however, Childress et al. refers to 'all other things being equal' as a form of measure (Childress et al. 2002). Allen and Selgelid (2017) interprets this as, all alternative options being equally effective, we ought to choose the option that is least costly. This could mean two things: (1) DCTA of choice is equally effective as the alternatives in achieving the end goal, i.e., contact tracing that can keep up with the rate of transmission; and (2) the extent to which one option impacts autonomy can be morally justified if it is the least morally costly option compared to other options which impact on individual autonomy to a greater extent. As discussed earlier, manual contact tracing alone is not a sufficient means for contact tracing in response to situations such as the Covid-19 pandemic. In this case, a comparison between manual and digital contact tracing methods will not be beneficial. What would be more useful is a comparison between the various types of DCTAs available. If all types of DCTAs are equally effective, a moral justification can be made for the types of DCTAs that are least costly to individual rights such as autonomy and informed consent. However, this too involves complexities which I will discuss below.

I have looked at the varying levels of effectiveness of centralized versus decentralized DCTAs and how the impact informed consent and autonomy. Decentralized data collection and storage poses challenges for health agencies, as decentralizing the data can negatively affect access to the data in the time it is needed. This is especially so for multi-agency responses. A centralized maximal approach is more effective as it provides readily available and accessible data. As a centralized maximal approach is more effective of the two methods, therefore meeting the condition of effectiveness, it would seem this option is in a better position to justify the use mandatory use of DCTAs. However, this option is more intrusive on privacy and does not provide much room for individual autonomy and informed consent compared to decentralized DCTAs. Therefore, while being the option for meeting the condition of effectiveness, it may not meet the condition of least infringement. The point I make here is this: mandatory use of DCTAs could possibly be justified under a public health ethics approach, based on the conditions that DCTAs are effective in achieving the intended outcomes (for this we need to have a clear understanding of the intended outcomes) and it is the least morally infringing option.

If the above conditions are met, there are additional factors such as morbidity and mortality which contribute to the justification for mandatory use of DCTAs as a public heath measure. There is an element of risk-based judgement in this type of justification.[10] What are the risks of disease spreading among the population? How

---

[10] The term 'risk' is defined as the possibility of experiencing a harm. Risk consists of two dimensions: (1) the magnitude or severity of the potential harm; and (2) the likelihood that this harm will occur. The significance of a risk depends on the interaction of these two considerations (Coleman 2021: 130–8).

many people are at risk of serious harm/injury or death? What level of burden would the outbreak place on healthcare services? Depending on a risk-based judgement, an argument could be made in defence of mandating some public health measures such as vaccination, restriction of free movement either in the form of lockdowns or isolation, and mandating that people wear personal protective equipment such as face masks. The justification here is that the benefits outweigh the risks. Extending this justification, it could be applied to the use of DCTAs as a necessary epidemiological tool. However, this is not a blanket justification. Risk and benefits are subjective to individual perception. For example, individuals who place a high value on privacy may consider unauthorized disclosure of personal information as troubling, while others who share information freely may not consider this as an issue. Similarly, how individuals perceive harm and benefits are both subjective to perception (Coleman 2021: 130–8).

Fairness in distribution of burdens is another reason that could be provided in defence of mandatory public health measures. Public health measures like any other collective measure, do not benefit everyone equally (Faden and Shebaya 2019). Some of the people within a given population stand to benefit very little from measures implemented at a population level, yet are required to follow mandatory measures that infringe on individual rights such as informed consent and autonomy. In this case, if there are no individual benefits to be gained an argument in favour of preserving these rights may seem plausible. However, there is another side to this perspective—some groups of people within a population may be at a greater risk or unfairly burdened by health risks. Consideration of fairness ought to apply in these situations. The moral justification here would be that burdens ought to be equivalent for everyone. Burdens here refer to health related burdens such as disease and disability and the burden of public health interventions. For example, vulnerable groups in a population such as the elderly, infants, and immunocompromised individuals are at greater risk from infectious diseases. Mandatory vaccination programs are a good example of this. Implemented at a population level, they serve two purposes, to protect the individual from acquiring a preventable disease, and to also protect the vulnerable. There is a moral justification and a legitimate argument in mandating healthy individuals to be vaccinated against a disease that poses a risk to the vulnerable population even if healthy individuals are not at risk (or the same level of risk) from the disease in question and may not stand to gain as much from vaccination.[11] Applying this analogy to mandatory use of DCTAs, we could expect individuals who have the

---

[11] For example, mandatory vaccination of healthy adults against Rubella to prevent the risk of Rubella passing to a foetus. In healthy adults, Rubella causes a skin rash and joint pain and does not present a significant risk, however, in a foetus, Rubella can cause birth defects, deafness, blindness, heart problems, brain damage, and has a high risk of death. Requiring healthy individuals to bear the burden of public health measures by mandatory vaccination against a disease that does not pose a great risk to them, could be morally justified to protect the vulnerable groups (foetus) who are at greater risk.

means and capacity to bear the burden, so that those in the population who are vulnerable and at greater risk are protected. It could be morally justified to mandate those who can, to use DCTAs even if it impacts autonomy and informed consent, so that the vulnerable groups in the population can be protected against risk of being infected.

An analysis of the two approaches; a bioethics and public health ethics approach, I propose that mandatory use of DCTAs could be justified under a public health ethics approach solely as a public health measure. However, even under the public health ethics approach, one that allows infringement of individual rights, this is not a blanket justification. It is justified under a very narrow set of circumstances and remains applicable as long as these narrow set of circumstances exist. Adam Henschke's chapter in this book provides a comprehensive discussion on this. I will address it briefly here.

First, the narrow justification rests on the state of emergency or extreme circumstances arising in a pandemic. I have proposed that the Covid-19 pandemic brought about a state of emergency on this scale. Several factors contribute to the proposition such as the significantly high morbidity and mortality rates, the rapid pace at which the disease spread, the lack of a known cure or treatment, and the burden on healthcare workers and infrastructure. Second, DCTAs as a public health measure would need to meet the justificatory conditions as put forward by Childress et al. and other proponents of public health ethics. I have discussed these justificatory conditions in the context of DCTAs, highlighting the possible complexities in relation to effectiveness and least infringement. Based on these factors, I propose that we ought to follow a public health ethics approach and that use of DCTAs could be morally justified within this narrow scope.

## Conclusion

As the Covid-19 pandemic unfolded, we saw an increase in the number of countries that used DCTAs as a public health measure. Some countries encouraged voluntary use of DCTAs while others mandated their use. In this chapter I looked at how DCTAs are being used and how this impacts an individual's right to informed consent and autonomy. I examined whether it is possible to achieve a balance between individual rights and the greater good of public health. This examination was based on two distinct approaches: a bioethics approach and a public health ethics approach. Mandatory use of DCTAs may not be morally justified under a strong bioethics perspective where informed consent and autonomy are among the core values. However, in responding to a pandemic the scale of Covid-19, an argument could be made against taking a bioethics approach and one in favour of a public health ethics approach. Based on public health ethics and the perspectives offered by ethicists such as O'Neill, Childress, Faden, and Selgelid, mandatory use of DCTA could be morally justified given it meets certain justifi-catory conditions such as necessity, effectiveness, and least infringement. This claim is not without caveats. Some DCTAs, whilst meeting one or two of the justificatory conditions, fail to meet all three conditions further complicating the matter. Other public health justifications provided in favour of mandatory use of DCTAs as a public good, consist of fairness in distributing health burdens and protecting vulnerable groups in the population. In the context of a pandemic such as Covid-19 where there is a significant level of risk and uncertainty, a defence in favour of mandatory use of DCTAs can be made. In this situation, we ought to follow a public health ethics approach until such time more is known, clarity is in our favour, and a better path identified.

# References

Allen, T. and M. J. Selgelid. 2017. 'Necessity and Least Infringement Conditions in Public Health Ethics'. *Medicine, Health Care, and Philosophy* 20 (4): 525–35.

Beauchamp, T. L. 2011. 'Informed Consent: Its History, Meaning, and Present Challenges', *Cambridge Quarterly of Healthcare Ethics* 20 (4): 515–23.

Beauchamp, T. L. and J. F. Childress. 2009. *Principles of Biomedical Ethics.* 6th edn.; New York: Oxford University Press; 99–120.

Beauchamp, T. L. and J. F. Childress. 2013. *Principles of Biomedical Ethics.* 7th edn.; New York: Oxford University Press; 99–138.

Bradford, L., M. Aboy, and K. Liddell. 2020. 'COVID-19 Contact Tracing Apps: A Stress Test for Privacy, the GDPR, and Data Protection Regimes'. *Journal of Law and the Biosciences* 7 (1).

Budin-Ljøsne, I. et al. 2017. 'Dynamic Consent: A Potential Solution to Some of the Challenges of Modern Biomedical Research'. *BMC Medical Ethics* 18 (1): 4–4.

Cattuto, C. and A. Spina. 2020. 'The Institutionalisation of Digital Public Health: Lessons Learned from the COVID-19 App'. *European Journal of Risk Regulation* 11 (2): 228–35.

Childress, J. F. et al. 2002. 'Public Health Ethics: Mapping the Terrain'. *The Journal of Law, Medicine & Ethics* 30 (2): 170–8.

Coleman, C. H. 2021. 'Risk-Benefit Analysis'. In *The Cambridge Handbook of Health Research Regulation* (Cambridge Law Handbooks), edited by Agomoni Ganguli-Mitra et al., 130–8. Cambridge: Cambridge University Press.

Danquah, L. O. et al. 2019. 'Use of a Mobile Application for Ebola Contact Tracing and Monitoring in Northern Sierra Leone: A Proof-Of-Concept Study'. *BMC Infectious Diseases* 19 (1): 810.

Dhar Chowdhury, S. and Oommen, A. M. 2020. 'Epidemiology of COVID-19', *Journal of Digestive Endoscopy*, 11 (01): 03–07.

Eyal, N. 2019. 'Informed Consent', in *The Stanford Encyclopedia of Philosophy* (Spring 2019 edn., edited by Edward N. Zalta. Metaphysics Research Lab, Stanford University.

Faden, R. R. and S. Shebaya. 2019. 'Public Health Programs and Policies: Ethical Justifications', in The Oxford Handbook of Public Health Ethics, 1 edn., edited by Anna C. Mastroianni, Jeffrey P. Kahn, and Nancy E. Kass. New York; Oxford University Press.

Goggin, G. 2020. 'COVID-19 Apps in Singapore and Australia: Reimagining Healthy Nations with Digital Technology'. *Media International Australia* 177 (1): 61–75.

Greenleaf, G. and Kemp, K. 2021. 'Police Access to COVID Check-in Data Is an Affront to Our Privacy. We Need Stronger and More Consistent Rules in Place'. *The Conversation.* https://theconversation.com/police-access-to-covid-check-in-data-is-an-affront-to-our-privacy-we-need-stronger-and-more-consistent-rules-in-place-167360, accessed 10 October 2021.

Henschke, A. 2017. *Ethics in an Age of Surveillance: Personal Information and Virtual Identities.* Cambridge; Cambridge University Press.

Henschke, A. 2018. 'Conceptualising Proportionality and Its Relation to Metadata'. In *Intelligence and the Function of Government*, edited by Daniel Baldino and Rhys Crawley. Carlton, Victoria: Melbourne University Press.

Hoffman, A. S. et al. 2020. 'Towards a Seamful Ethics of Covid-19 Contact Tracing Apps?', *Ethics and Information Technology.*

Jacob, S. and J. Lawarée. 2021. 'The Adoption of Contact Tracing Applications of Covid-19 by European Governments'. *Policy Design and Practice* 4 (1): 44–58.

Johansson, M. A. et al. 2021. 'SARS-CoV-2 Transmission from People without Covid-19 Symptoms'. *JAMA Network Open* 4 (1): e2035057.

Kahn, J., ed. 2020. *Digital Contact Tracing for Pandemic Response: Ethics and Governance Guidance.* Baltimore; Johns Hopkins University Press.

Lodders, A. and J. M. Paterson. 2020. 'Scrutinising COVIDSafe: Frameworks for Evaluating Digital Contact Tracing Technologies'. *Alternative Law Journal* 45 (3): 153–61.

Maccari, L. and V. Cagno. 2021. 'Do We Need a Contact Tracing App?'. *Computer Communications* 166: 9–18.

Miller, S. 2014. 'Joint Actions, Social Institutions and Collective Goods: A Teleological Account'. In *Institutions, Emotions, and Group Agents: Contributions to Social Ontology*, edited by Anita Konzelmann Ziv and Hans Bernhard Schmid, 99–115. Dordrecht: Springer Netherlands.

Miller, S. and M. Smith. 2021. 'Ethics, Public Health and Technology Responses to COVID-19'. *Bioethics* 35 (4): 366–71.

Murray, J. and A. L. Cohen. 2017. 'Infectious Disease Surveillance'. *International Encyclopedia of Public Health* 2 (4): 222–9.

Nuffield Council on Bioethics. 2007. *Public Health: Ethical Issues.* London: Cambridge Publishers Ltd.

O'Neill, O. 2004. 'Informed consent and public health', *Philosophical transactions. Biological sciences*, 359 (1447): 1133–36.

Park, M. et al. 2020. 'A Systematic Review of Covid-19 Epidemiology Based on Current Evidence'. *Journal of Clinical Medicine*, 9 (4): 967.

Parker, M. J. et al. 2020. 'Ethics of Instantaneous Contact Tracing Using Mobile Phone Apps in the Control of the Covid-19 Pandemic'. *Journal of Medical Ethics* 46 (7): 427–31.

Pollock, A. M. and J. Lancaster. 2020. 'Asymptomatic Transmission of Covid-19'. *BMJ*, m4851.

Powers, M. and R. Faden. 2013. 'Social Practices, Public Health and the Twin Aims of Justice: Responses to Comments'. *Public Health Ethics* 6 (1): 45–9.

Powers, M., R. Faden, and Y. Saghai. 2012. 'Liberty, Mill and the Framework of Public Health Ethics'. *Public Health Ethics* 5 (1): 6–15.

Ryan, M. 2020. 'In defence of digital contact-tracing: human rights, South Korea and Covid-19', *International journal of pervasive computing and communications*, 16 (4): 383–407.

Steinsbekk, K. S., B. Kåre Myskja, and B. Solberg. 2013. 'Broad Consent versus Dynamic Consent in Biobank Research: Is Passive Participation an Ethical Problem?', *European Journal of Human Genetics: EJHG* 21 (9): 897–902.

Storeng, K. T. and A. de Bengy Puyvallée. 2021. 'The Smartphone Pandemic: How Big Tech and Public Health Authorities Partner in the Digital Response to Covid-19', *Global Public Health* 16 (8–9): 1482–98.

Thomas Craig, K. J. et al. 2021. 'Effectiveness of Contact Tracing for Viral Disease Mitigation and Suppression: Evidence-Based Review'. *JMIR Public Health and Surveillance* 7 (10): e32468.

White, L. and P. van Basshuysen. 2021a. 'Privacy versus Public Health? A Reassessment of Centralised and Decentralised Digital Contact Tracing'. *Science and Engineering Ethics* 27 (2): 23.

White, L. and P. van Basshuysen. 2021b. 'Without a Trace: Why Did Corona Apps Fail?'. *Journal of Medical Ethics*. medethics-2020-107061.

World Health Organization. 2022. Coronavirus (COVID-19) Dashboard. Geneva, Switzerland.

Wymant, C., et al. 2021. 'The Epidemiological Impact of the NHS Covid-19 App'. *Nature (London)* 594 (7863): 408–12.

# 8

# Surveillance, Democracy, and Protest in a Time of Climate Crisis

*Katerina Hadjimatheou*

The question of how political protest should be regulated and policed in a democracy has long been a topic of philosophical debate (Rawls, 1999, Brownlee, 2012). But it has acquired renewed political urgency in recent years. Most recently, government responses to the Covid-19 pandemic have prompted public protests across the world, often in defiance of strict lockdown restrictions enacted under emergency legislation. These have ranged from anti-vax demonstrations contesting the introduction of restrictions to the activities of the non-vaccinated, to demonstrations related to the economic consequences of the pandemic, to protests against the methods adopted by law enforcement in their efforts to police lockdowns. In some cases, pandemic-related protest groups have also sought to coincide their actions with demonstrations organized by more established campaign groups, such as climate change activists, in order to draw attention to their cause.[1] This chapter examines the question of how surveillance should be used to police protest in a time of emergency, focusing on environmental activism as a case study from which conclusions relevant to protests in other conditions of crisis can be drawn.[2]

A growing acknowledgement of a global climate emergency has propelled the rise of environmental protest movements such as Extinction Rebellion (ER), Fridays for Future, and Global Climate Strike (Kyllonen 2014). The approach of such movements is to invite mass participation in non-violent but often disruptive protest or 'actions', such as using passive resistance to block key roads in cities in order to draw attention to climate change. Extinction Rebellion also seek to prompt political change, both by influencing government policy, and by advocating the

---

[1] In 2021 anti-vax protesters in London appeared to highjack Extinction Rebellion gatherings, sparking violence which led to the injury of four police officers (BBC 2021).

[2] Note that there is also a pertinent distinction between the two groups as well. While most today would endorse the right of both groups to protest, contemporary society is generally more sympathetic to environmental protest than to anti-vaccine protestors. This may lead to important considerations regarding when surveillance may be used to legitimately deter activists from engaging in illegal activities, such as protesting outside schools or the 6 January storming of the US Capitol. While these considerations are important to the overall debate, they go beyond the scope of this current chapter which focuses on police surveillance of legitimate protest.

Katerina Hadjimatheou, *Surveillance, Democracy, and Protest in a Time of Climate Crisis* In: *The Ethics of Surveillance in Times of Emergency.* Edited by: Kevin Macnish and Adam Henschke, Oxford University Press.
© Oxford University Press 2023. DOI: 10.1093/oso/9780192864918.003.0009

establishment of 'citizens' assemblies', to which they argue climate policy decisions should be delegated.[3] While ER's campaign for citizens' assemblies has yet to yield results, there is already significant evidence showing that mass climate protests have been successful on a range of other important fronts, including by increasing public support for climate change action (Bugden 2020), prompting regional governments to reduce emissions locally (Muñoz et al. 2018), and convincing firms to divest in fossil fuels resulting in emissions reductions (Glomsrød and Wei 2018).[4]

The rationale and rhetoric of emergencies is actively deployed by environmental groups seeking to justify the disruption to daily life caused by their protests. For example, Extinction Rebellion defend their campaigns by emphasizing the existential stakes of climate change and stressing the need for exceptional measures that reach, in their words, 'beyond politics'. ER's case for replacing policymaking by representative democracy with a deliberative alternative is similarly based on the argument that climate change has proven to be a challenge 'too controversial and difficult for politicians to deal with successfully by themselves' given the pressures of the electoral cycle and the political influence of lobbyists representing polluting industries (Extinction Rebellion 2019a). Their position is both supported and contradicted by the fact that, at least in the UK, where ER was founded, Parliament has recognized officially the existence of a climate emergency and appears likely to pass new legislation authorizing the use of emergency powers in response.[5] Political acknowledgment of an ecological emergency has also begun to influence judicial decision-making around the criminality of 'direct action', or acts of civil disobedience undertaken by environmental protesters. In 2021, the convictions of three ER protesters were overturned by a judge who found that blocking a public highway was a proportionate exercise of the right to protest peacefully (Casciani 2021).

In contrast, the approach of law enforcement to environmental protest in the UK has recently hardened, with police announcing intentions to 'rebalance' enforcement in favour of business and daily life, and against protesters seeking to disrupt these (HMICFRS 2021; NPCC 2022). Some evidence of a toughening of the police stance is already evident: in 2021 London police exercised powers designed for the prevention of serious crime and terrorism to raid an architecture studio storing scaffolding that had been used by some ER protesters. Once inside, they seized the mobile phones and laptops of those present for inspection and arrested them on suspicion of 'conspiracy to create a public nuisance'. Police have also begun to use less orthodox methods such as 'doxxing' to shame protesters. For example, in 2021 London's MET police posted on Facebook the names and addresses of climate

---

[3] For a discussion of ER and the 'securitization' of climate change see Slaven and Hayden (2020).
[4] For a summary of recent research in this field, see Fisher and Nasrin (2020).
[5] Climate and Ecological Bill 2021–22.

protesters involved in peaceful disruption of a printing press, which led to their harassment by members of the public (APPG 2021: para.156[e]).

Police in England and Wales have also declared an intention to intensify their use of surveillance powers against protest movements, through the use of informants[6] and undercover police infiltrators and the expansion of technological surveillance such as facial recognition (HMICFRS 2021: 2). A recent national review recommends police urgently improve their intelligence about individual protesters 'who seek to bring about political or social change in a way that involves unlawful behaviour or criminality' in order to prevent or disrupt them. At the same time, new legislation currently making its way through Parliament lowers the threshold at which police action to prevent or disperse a public protest is legally justified, making it easier for surveillance to be deployed in support of such measures (Home Office 2021).

These developments invite a re-examination of the ethics of police surveillance of protest movements. Environmental and climate activism serves as a useful case study in this regard. While environmental movements are by no means the only protest groups subject to police surveillance, their broad reach and ability to generate mass participation, including amongst children (an estimated 7.6 million people participated in climate strikes across the world in 2019 [Rosane 2019]) means that climate activists are more likely to come under such surveillance than others. Environmental protest movements are only likely to expand their following further as climate-related disasters and crises increase in both frequency and severity, touching the lives of ever greater numbers of people. Finally, the fact that government actions continue to fall short of what climate science has identified as necessary to avert catastrophic effects suggests that public protest will continue to have a key political role to play on this issue. For these reasons, issues around police surveillance of protest movements are intertwined with urgent political questions about how prepared we are as democratic societies to deal with a climate emergency, an emergency that intersects ever more frequently with other crises, including the ongoing Covid-19 pandemic.

## The Ethics of Police Surveillance of Protest: Privacy and the Chilling Effect

Most people's experience of exercising the right to protest[7] is conditioned by how broadly or narrowly that right is interpreted by police, and by the intrusiveness of

---

[6] Evidence of ongoing police attempts to recruit environmental activists as informants can be found, e.g., on Netpol's website and the APPG report (para.156[b]).
[7] The right to protest is recognized as a discrete legal right in the European convention of human rights, include freedom of assembly, association, and expression.

the means used by police to enforce its boundaries.[8] Police in many countries have broad discretion to interpret where thresholds of legality lie and to choose which tactics—from persuasion to 'kettling',[9] water cannon or tear gas—to use to contain or disperse protests.[10] Discussions of the ethics of police surveillance of political activity have tended to focus on the risk it poses to the rights of the individual (Baker et al. 2017). But, as sociolegal theorists Starr et al. (2008) and Aston (2017) have argued, police surveillance also affects protest movements as collectives. People tend to exercise their right to protest through a movement, group, or organization, and not alone standing on a soapbox. Indeed, for most people involved in activism, a protest movement is both an important stimulus for the formation of a political stance and a forum within which to express political views and be heard. For this reason, protest movements should be understood as vital prerequisites to the exercise of those rights, contributing directly to the capacity of individuals to exercise those rights (or, put otherwise, facilitating the conversion of formal freedoms to protest into 'capabilities' to do so). The existence and operation of such groups cannot be reduced to aggregate exercises of individual rights. So an examination of the impact of police surveillance on protest must include an examination of its effects on those groups. Specifically, it must examine the impact on groups' ability to 'mobilise' for action, with mobilization understood in sociological terms as processes of building support and planning activities, for example through 'meetings, networks, strategic planning, and extensive communicative and solidarity building activity' (Starr 2008: 257).

Both Starr and Aston make important contributions in this respect, drawing on first-hand testimonies of activists who have been subject to police surveillance to demonstrate empirically the considerable ways in which it stunts and inhibits the mobilization of protest movements. While Starr provides a general overview of all kinds of state surveillance on a broad range of social justice protest movements, Aston focuses exclusively on the effects of overt—i.e., publicly visible—police surveillance on environmental activism in the UK. Taken together, their insights advance current understandings of the implications of police surveillance in important ways, in particular by providing a deeper and more systematic account of how police surveillance exerts a 'chilling effect' on the collective exercise of

---

[8] This merely restates political scientist Bayley's insight that the way in which police exercise discretion 'directly affects the reality of freedom' for citizens (Bayley 1985: 5).

[9] A controversial police tactic that involves corralling protesters into contained areas, often for hours without food or water or means of departure. When protesters are permitted to leave the kettle, this is typically through a single point of exit where police subject them to questioning and search.

[10] As a recent parliamentary review noted, when police are given expanded coercive powers in relation to authorizing protest, they become both 'law maker' and 'law enforcer' (APPG 2021). This undermines their legitimacy as normatively neutral enforcers of legislation. What is more, it allows the significant reasons police have to want to discourage, prevent and constrain assemblies (mainly resource considerations as discussed in footnote 3 above) to shape illegitimately their determination of whether a protest is legal.

political liberties. In doing so, both aim to lay the conceptual ground for better informed judicial assessments of the proportionality, and thereby the legality, of specific tactics of protest policing.

The present chapter builds on this body of work in two ways. First, by extending the analysis to examine in depth the distinctive effects of a specific kind of surveillance known as 'covert human intelligence' (or more commonly undercover infiltration), on protest movement mobilization. Second, by proposing refinements to the concept of 'chill' in order to capture more precisely the impact of surveillance on the ability of protest movements to address social problems. The aim of the discussion to follow is therefore twofold: to understand better the practices and tactics police deploy to surveil contemporary protest movements, and to conceptualize more precisely their impact. The first section addresses the first of these aims by providing an overview of police surveillance as documented in reliable accounts drawn from four kinds of sources: testimony from two activists (referred to as Luke and Davin) interviewed by the author as part of an ongoing study of police surveillance and the chilling effect;[11] activist testimony as reported in previous articles by Starr et al. (2008), Aston (2017), and Gilmore et al. (2020); evidence and statements submitted by activists, their lawyers, and police for public inquiry into undercover policing currently in progress in the UK; and a 2020 parliamentary report on the policing of public protest. A distinction is made between overt and covert surveillance. The second section focuses on the concept of chill.

## Police Surveillance of Protest Movements: Tactics and Practices

### *Overt* Surveillance during Protests and Assemblies and Immediately before and after Them

Overt police surveillance of protests is justified by police as a form of intelligence gathering; to enable them to identify anyone who breaks the law should the protest turn into disorder; and to identify those with organizational and leadership roles in a movement. Monitoring can involve searches, questioning, filming, and photographing of all and any protesters, but also more intense, targeted surveillance of specific activists identified as leaders. A 2019 court case revealed that police use data collected at protests to compile databases and detailed dossiers on activists, even those who have never been even distantly associated with

[11] This study, part of the Human Rights, Big Data, and Technology project, is funded by the Economic and Social Research Council under Grant ES/M010236/1. Interviews were carried out in London in 2019. Participants were recruited in collaboration with the civil liberties organization Liberty. Ethical approval was granted by the University of Essex Research Ethics Committee. Quotes from activist research participants cited below are referred to by their pseudonyms Luke and Davin.

criminality.[12] Though police justify the use of these kinds of surveillance powers as a means of identifying and disrupting protesters who are violent and intent on criminality, in practice they tend to be directed towards everyone present at a protest, including those clearly identified as legal observers, medics, and journalists (APPG 2021: paras. 148–9). Recent years have also seen the use of more aggressive techniques of registering and monitoring protesters. In 2013, police were found by a judge to have illegally 'kettled' large numbers of protesters into a small area and then obliged them to provide their personal details, submit to a search, and be filmed and photographed as a condition of release (Mengesha v Commissioner of Police of the Metropolis: 2013).[13]

Activists described the impact of these kinds of indiscriminate data gathering as exerting a deterrence or 'chilling' effect on the exercise of political freedoms by discouraging people from participating in protest. In addition to the unpleasantness of being 'kettled' and treated as suspicious by police, which most would reasonably want to avoid, some people have an insecure immigration status and fear detention or deportation if the police label them as criminal in an official database (Aston 2017: 4); some may be on probation or other restriction orders and fear re-criminalization; and some may fear racism, brutality and disproportionate criminalization from the police because they or people who share their racial or other traits have done so in the past (Starr et al. 2008: 258–9). In the UK, fears of being included in police databases are also linked to recent revelations that police shared personal details of environmental activists and union organizers with private companies which compiled blacklists of people who were then excluded from employment, in some cases for decades (Lubbers 2012: ch. 2).[14]

During protests, police routinely target intense surveillance at specific activists who have presumably been identified as leaders or instigators of protests. A distinctive tactic of police appears to be singling out individual activists and calling to them by name, with the individuals concerned having no idea how police had identified them. One activist reports that this occurred 'all the time … shouting from vans, the other side of crowds, pointing me out in a way that made it clear that the aim was to make me know I was being watched' (Jeremy, quoted in Aston 2017: 8, see also Gilmore 2020: 371). Another described this tactic as 'pure intimidation' (ibid.). In addition, many activists reported being closely tailed and

---

[12] Similarly, in 2019 a court found that police had been systematically monitoring and recording information about peaceful protesters simply because they attended protest events. In the specific case that prompted the trial, an elderly protester discovered that police had included detailed information on him in a database of 'domestic extremists' without any ground for suspicion of criminality (Catt vs United Kingdom 2019).

[13] A 'sneaky' use of powers allowing police to search people for possession of weapons under counter-terrorism laws was also used to obtain identifying information from activists (Bob, quoted in Aston 2017: 7, see also p. 6).

[14] A collection of journalistic reports on blacklisting is available here: https://www.hazards.org/blacklistblog/

photographed and filmed by police, before, during and sometimes long after protests. Thus, one spoke for many when he talked of having 'one or two uniformed police following you, wherever you go, whatever you do' (Jack, quoted in Aston 2017: 7). This was described as intrusive and frightening. It also induced in activists a preoccupation with police, which one described as having police 'infiltrating your way of thinking' (Brian, quoted in Gilmore et al. 2020: 372). Similarly, another activist who had been followed constantly for four days was left feeling that surveillance had 'taken over [his] life' as he found himself thinking and even dreaming about police all the time (John, quoted in Aston 2017: 8).

These testimonies draw attention to the expressive and indeed performative aspects of this kind of surveillance. Intense, targeted surveillance conveys a message to specific activists that police consider them troublemakers and will not leave them alone until they stop participating in activism. But it also shows people at the margins of protest movements that the authorities consider those at the centre to be dangerous and criminal, thus, in the words of one activist 'put [ting] people off from wanting to participate' (Jenny, quoted in Aston 2017: 4, 11). For example, one activist in Aston's study reported that an old acquaintance of his told him that she 'didn't really want to associate with me' after she saw him being surrounded by uniformed police during a protests, who were constantly taking 'large numbers of photographs from a very short distance'. The acquaintance told him that '[s]he was scared she'd be targeted in a similar manner or worse' (Evan, quoted in Aston 2017: 4, 11). This speaks to the ways police surveillance undermines the ability of protest groups to attract and retain members.

The chilling effect exerted by this kind of police surveillance was also described as creating fear or suspicion within movements, chilling associations between existing members and helping to create schisms. As one activist reported, 'sometimes their presence, which is supposedly to monitor and prevent... is quite divisive and creates this kind of "that's the militant people over there, with the cameras", and other people are drawn away from that, because why would you want to be [associated]?' (Jenny, quoted in Aston 2017: 11). A further way in which police surveillance divided groups was by prompting activists already under heavy surveillance to isolate themselves during protests, in order to protect more peripheral protesters from unwanted police attention. For example, one of Aston's participants reported that police would immediately stop and search anyone who approached her, so that she felt forced both to avoid social interaction during protest—thereby risking seeming unfriendly and aloof—and 'to warn other people that that was the consequence of associating with us on a protest... [that] police will take an interest in you' (Ellen, quoted in Aston 2017: 4). Similarly, another described how, when police 'were following me, personally, around on demonstrations, I would end up on my own... because I wouldn't want people to be with me [and] people also don't want to be around you' (Esther, quoted in Aston 2017: 7).

## Surveillance of Non-Protest Gatherings: Meetings, Camps, Workshops, Etc.

Away from protests themselves, environmental activists describe a pattern of heavy overt police surveillance of meetings, in one case every single meeting that took place over a period of two years (Magnus, quoted in Aston 2017: 10). This typically involved numerous uniformed officers with clearly marked vehicles stationed directly outside the venue, filming and taking photographs of every person entering and leaving the building so that, in the words of one activist interviewed for this chapter, 'there's no way of getting in or out of the building without being filmed' (Davin). Activists believed police used this kind of monitoring to build an intelligence picture of the organization and individual members through 'profile-building, you know, who turns up at these same different events, who's involved' (ibid.). But they also felt it was used expressively, 'to intimidate people' and to deter newcomers from becoming involved in the movement by sending a message to the effect that 'if you even want to *talk* to these people about what they are doing, you're on file. We have four officers taking this down, that's how seriously we are taking this' (Magnus, quoted in Aston 2017: 10).

Activists both in the UK and the US were convinced that this strategy was successful in deterring people from getting involved in activism. One participant spoke for many when he said that people 'who had seemed quite confident and really excited and enthused about getting involved in the movement would come to a meeting and they'd suddenly shrink, and be less confident and they would not participate and often they didn't come back' (Ricky, quoted in Aston 2017: 11). This hampered the ability of groups to engage new members. It also demoralized existing members: as one US activist explained 'people are staying home to avoid being on a list, so then it feels like nobody cares' (Starr et al. 2008: 259). Activists in Starr et al.'s study felt that a heavy police presence at meetings 'sullies the reputation of organizations' (Starr et al. 2008: 265), tainting them as criminal and leading other organizations using the same venue to view them with hostility, with some venue owners refusing to rent them space for their meetings, further hampering efforts to organize (ibid. 259). More generally, overt police surveillance was felt to tarnish activism as a means of political expression, and thus alienate people from the desire to become involved in activism. As one of Starr et al.'s participants said, 'even the word "activist" is stigmatized. People have disgust for what you do. You're not a committed, responsible citizen' (Starr 2008: 264).

Activists also reported overt surveillance of other non-protest gatherings such as workshops, festivals and camps, designed to generate new ideas and build social capital and solidarity. In 2008 a climate camp in the UK was surrounded by 1400 police officers, a number that almost equalled that of activists (Saunders and Price 2009: 118). Those entering and leaving were subjected routinely to stops and searches, resulting for some participants in several searches a day (Schlembach 2018: 501). Participants in Aston's study emphasized again the expressive aspect of this kind of police monitoring. For example, one activist at a women's peace camp described how sometimes police would arrive suddenly at night 'with cameras, they video everyone. From quite close, within a few feet' (Iona, quoted in Aston 2017: 112), while another at an environmental camp described police as a constant presence, 'sitting in the bushes taking pictures of people eating, having discussions, in workshops' and even monitoring the open toilet facilities (Ricki, quoted in Aston 2018: 112). This apparently intentionally conspicuous police monitoring disrupted mobilization in two ways: by ruining the sense of a space of solidarity where interactions were spontaneous and ideas could be explored and expressed safely, and by creating a collective preoccupation with police surveillance.

The preoccupation described here mirrors the individual fixation with police surveillance described by activists who were singled out for monitoring, but at a collective level. In one case, this preoccupation was described as derailing the focus of an entire event, shifting collective attention away from climate change and towards questions of how to manage police surveillance. One activist described how police would arrive, periodically but at unpredictable times and without warning, to a climate festival, demanding immediate tours of the site ostensibly to check compliance with rules on health and safety and trespass. He says:

> they started off by just having two officers walk round with somebody, and then they wanted three and then they wanted to make it more frequent. They would just turn up with more, they would turn up and say 'we want to do it now. And if you don't let us check that everything's alright we will have to assume the worst and you won't like it', basically threats to bust on site and close down the camp. And . . . we'd have to stop the meetings . . . we'd have to break and say, 'do we let them on, do we let them on more?    (Magnus, quoted in Aston 2018: 179)

The testimonies discussed in this section challenge current police and legal conceptualizations of surveillance as a kind of passive 'monitoring' or mere 'gathering of intelligence' by showing how they constitute an active, expressive, and sometimes even performative means of deterring and disrupting peaceful political activity.

## Undercover Policing: Infiltration

In 2010, it was revealed that since 1968, 150 British undercover police had infiltrated over 1000 peaceful environmental, social justice, and left-wing political groups.[15] Undercover officers lived with activists for years, some had long-term intimate relationships with unsuspecting women (including in a small number of cases, fathering children), and all collected vast banks of detailed information on anyone associated with the groups. As the many testimonies of activists and even undercover agents themselves now reveal, infiltration also involved police stepping into key organizational roles in political movements: taking positions on national executive committees, as treasurers, drafting manuals used by protesters, running logistics for protest camps, and so on.[16] This enabled police to collect information on membership and finances, to obtain keys to buildings and passwords to email inboxes, and to be party to all plans for political action.

While it is impossible to assess precisely the impact of undercover infiltration on the ability of movements to mobilize, there is evidence that police sought to disrupt, divide, and discredit organizations from the inside.[17] Documents submitted to the public inquiry detail how officers used their senior positions 'to discredit others within the organization and assist in sowing discord' (ibid.: 10), for example, by lobbying to have other senior members of committees removed and in one case even planning to overthrow and replace the leadership of the organization.[18] At least some used their position to 'sabotage the organization' and actively disrupt organizational activities, for example by deploying their advance knowledge of the locations of public meetings 'to enable uniformed officers to warn the proprietors (falsely) that the organization was illegal'. The venues 'were encouraged to cancel the meetings' (Opening Statement to the Undercover Policing Inquiry on behalf of Lois Austin et al. 2020: 9). In one now notorious case, an officer was instructed to infiltrate a family campaign seeking justice for a victim of a racist murder which the police had failed to investigate properly. The aim was to try to find information with which to smear and discredit the family and their campaign (Evans and Lewis 2013). Undercover officers also advocated for and indeed coordinated acts of illegality, apparently in order to divide groups and delegitimize them in the eyes of the public (Evans and Lewis 2012). In one example, an officer proposed repeatedly to activists that their organization, which

---

[15] These figures are gathered from a range of sources submitted to the ongoing Undercover Policing Inquiry and cannot be attributed to a single source.

[16] This strategy was acknowledged in the witness statement of an undercover officer to the ongoing public inquiry (First Witness Statement of HN301 2019: 6). And it is now in the public domain that many undercover officers including Mark Kennedy, 'Vince Miller', 'Rick Gibson', 'Carlo Neri', 'Marco Jacobs', and others held organizational roles. For example, 'Gary Roberts', who enrolled as a student in his undercover role, became vice president of the student union.

[17] The counterfactual estimations would involve too many assumptions to be reliable. But the fact that police sought roles that otherwise would have been taken by genuine activists is itself likely to have had a distorting effect on the strategies pursued. Activists have claimed that their activities 'influenced the political direction of' of organizations such as Greenpeace (Opening Submissions 2020: 20–1).

[18] 'Rick Gibson' is mentioned repeatedly as seeking to create rifts within the organization he had infiltrated and taken a leading role within (Undercover Policing Inquiry Tranche 1 [Phase 2] Evidence Hearings, Day 10 transcript, pp. 80–5).

had never used violence before, should firebomb a shop, apparently in full knowledge that 'provocation of serious criminality would not just discredit organizations, it would destroy them' (Opening Statement to Undercover Policing Inquiry 1: 18). Here we can see how police surveillance goes well beyond passive monitoring and intelligence gathering of protest movements, to include active manipulation and disruption. Surveillance techniques are used for interference rather than (merely) insight.

A different way in which undercover infiltration disrupts protest movements from within is by provoking their adoption of what is known as 'security culture'. Security culture refers to the adoption of organizational measures, behaviours—including language—and attitudes designed to defend and protect a group against surveillance and infiltration. Security culture remains almost entirely unexamined in the academic literature on undercover policing or surveillance of protest movements. A notable exception is Starr et al., who discuss it only briefly, mentioning that it hobbles organizations by leading them to plan and carry out even basic organizational activities in secret, but also that it poisons them by encouraging pervasive mutual suspicion, divisions between those who have proven their credentials and those who have not, and active distrust of new arrivals (Starr et al. 2008: 263). Starr et al.'s findings were echoed by a UK activist interviewed for the chilling effect study who explained:

> it's how you interact with new people in activism, are they undercover, can you trust them, it's awful because it creates a false paranoia in circles which you think should be safe and, you know, caring. You're working together with likeminded individuals to make a change to the environment . . . as opposed to bad things like terrorism.

As we will now see, for some activists, security culture has been the single most damaging consequence of police surveillance for protest movements.

Above, it was argued that surveillance can have the effect of fixating the attention of individuals and groups on policing and surveillance to the detriment of organization and mobilization. Undercover infiltration, or the widespread awareness of the possibility of it, has a similar effect, causing organizations to devote time, attention, and organizational resources to security and to prioritize it over issues of vital importance such as recruitment, egalitarianism inclusiveness, solidarity and community building, and efficiency. For example, one activist interviewed for this chapter described having

> constant debates about which email system and messaging apps are secure, using poorly designed platforms and switching all the time . . . it has affected our movement because a lot of people think [we're using] a shit platform . . . every collective has this discussion, the extent to which security culture is used in their

organizational structure, so the same conversations happen again and again ... it really messes with people's heads.   (Davin)

Security culture was described as both constraining and distorting communication and association within groups, with frank conversations happening only in selected fora and only after all those present have been subject to background checks or 'vouched for'. As a veteran environmental activist interviewed for this chapter explained:

> you're thinking are they from a private company or from the authorities? You have to try and do your research about them without offending them and that takes time, it has to be done very carefully, because I'm sure as many tactics as activists come up with, there's countermeasures—especially with all this new technology of state surveillance to come round that make fake IDs and fake profiles. You have to challenge, that's the kind of level of work you have to do, you go to their family home, meet their mother, their father, you know is this person who they say they are, you know it's kind of horrible.   (Luke)

He described how being vouched for is also a condition of being included in meetings: 'you arrive at a meeting and before it starts you say "is everybody here comfortable with who is present? Or "put up your hand if you can vouch for this person so we can make sure we're all vouched for" ... These precautionary things, it leaves a very uncomfortable feeling in meetings sometimes.' As will be discussed in the following section, these organizational reactions to surveillance are quite distinct from mere inhibition or self-censorship typically associated with fear of being monitored.

Both of the activists interviewed for this chapter were convinced that security culture had fundamentally corrupted and disrupted previously peaceful, united movements, with one saying, 'all those years of infiltration had a huge effect on bringing distrust, inhibited and restricted us in so many ways ... the amount of people the movement has lost from being distrustful, unfriendly', and another adding: 'security cannot be at the expense of a mass movement, and it has paralysed groups' (Davin and Luke, respectively). There is an obvious irony in the fact that protest movements have sought to protect themselves from unwanted police surveillance by developing their own surveillance techniques and turning these on each other. But there is also something deeply ironic about the way police can induce peaceful, lawful campaigns for social and environmental justice to behave as if they were clandestine, criminal organizations with something to hide, just by treating them as if they were such.

This section has sought to draw attention to the array of ways in which police surveillance of political movements inhibits, disrupts, and distorts the exercise of political freedoms to protest. Though activists have attempted to raise awareness of these implications in various forums,[19] they remain entirely unacknowledged by police, whose official guidance only requires them to consider the impact of their actions on individual rights. They are also overlooked in recent public discussion of the ethics of undercover policing, which has focused overwhelmingly on issues arising in relation to officers' intimate relationships with female activists. The absence of debate about—and indeed legal recognition of—this distinctive category of harms or wrongs reflects the lack of an accepted vocabulary or concept with which to describe it. The next section addresses this gap.

## Conceptualizing the Impact of Surveillance on Protest Mobilization: The Limits of the 'Chilling Effect'

While Starr et al. and Gilmore et al. limit themselves to identifying and describing the implications of police surveillance, Aston conceptualizes them and in doing so makes an important step towards refining and deepening ethical and legal debate on this topic. Her argument is that surveillance practices 'create harms that extend beyond individual privacy, by "chilling" the process of assembly mobilizations and amounting to (at least arguably) a restriction of assembly rights' (Aston 2018: 34–5). Like legal theorists before her, Aston understands the chilling effect as deterrence of benign, worthy, or legally protected behaviour, resulting from ambiguities or uncertainties in the law or its application (Schauer 1978; Kendrick 2013; Pech 2021). This notion of chill has been used in empirical efforts to demonstrate the causal relationship between mass surveillance of online communications and self-censoring behaviour by writers, activists, and citizens in general (Penney 2016; Stoycheff et al. 2020; PEN 2015). Thus chill is a kind of externality (or unintended but costly byproduct) of uncertainty and latent threat: people are unsure of whether or at what point their exercise of protected behaviours will invite negative consequences, therefore they protect themselves by refraining from those behaviours. According to this account, chilling effects may not necessarily constitute direct interferences with rights, but they reduce the scope of their free exercise (typically beyond what is justified or legitimate) and this is problematic in a liberal democracy (ibid.). Aston's contribution to this line of legal theorizing about chill is both to extend it to police surveillance of environmental activism, and to expand it to include effects on organizations—in this case protest movements—alongside individuals.

This 'classic' theory of chill has advanced significantly our understanding of the inhibiting and disruptive impacts of police surveillance, and their moral

---

[19] See, for example, the Charter for Freedom of Assembly Rights, devised by the association of protest groups Netpol (Network for Police Monitoring) which has been signed by forty-four different groups in the UK.

implications. But there are three features of it that limit its ability to capture the full range of inhibiting and disruptive impacts on protest movements described above. These are: its insistence on uncertainty as a causal factor; its recognition of only one motivating attitude, namely fear of negative consequence; and its reductive assumption that outcomes are limited to individuals *refraining from* certain behaviours. Taken together, these conditions exclude many of the effects this chapter—and Aston herself—wishes to draw attention to. For example, the conspicuous overt police monitoring at protest camps Aston describes was unambiguous in its scope and aims, and hardly provoked fear in activists. Though it did inhibit free and frank discussion to some extent, it was primarily disruptive, diverting activists' attention and resources towards talking, thinking about, and managing police surveillance. Similar points can be made about the development of security culture in protest movements: here, uncertainty about infiltration was key, but the effect was not only to inhibit behaviours but also to generate *new* self-protective behaviours that were themselves deleterious to the movement. In contrast, Penney (2016) and Stoycheff et al.'s (2020) studies of online surveillance recognize only the 'silencing' or 'avoidance' effects of chill. A more nuanced concept of chill than that provided by the 'classic' theory is therefore required.

In his deep and wide-ranging analysis of the chilling effect, legal theorist Penney (forthcoming) draws both on the social theory of privacy and on social scientific insights into the effects of surveillance on behaviour to argue for an expansion of the concept of chill in a way that 'take[s] the social shaping of the *subject* of chilling effects seriously'. His 'social conformity theory of chilling effects' expands the definition of chilled behaviour to include 'speaking, acting, or doing, just in a way that conforms to, or is in compliance with, a perceived social norm' (2022: 5). He also rightly does away with the uncertainty criterion in relation to chilling effects of state surveillance, pointing out that chill can occur even in conditions in which activists know their activism will result in them being watched, followed, recorded and categorized, and ultimately suffering interference with their liberties. Penney's theory constitutes an important step towards recognizing that surveillance not only deters people from acting in certain ways but also conditions and distorts their motivations and preferences. This enables his theory to accommodate the way heavy overt police surveillance may lead third party observers to associate activism with bad and criminal behaviour and therefore to adapt their preferences around the exercise of their political freedoms to protest (though he does not explicitly note this himself).

However, like legal theorists before him, Penney ultimately specifies the behavioural outcomes in a way that is too narrow. As the examples given above illustrate, a desire to avoid legal, privacy or other harms associated with state surveillance can lead to a range of behaviours beyond mere conformity, such as actions designed to avoid surveillance, to manage it, to conceal behaviour, or to obstruct or counteract it. His theory neither explains nor captures these important behaviours. At the same time, Penney's theory is too expansive: by including *any* kind of threat of sanction from any source, and conformity with *any* perceived social norm, it loses sight of the distinctive moral problem with chill (and indeed the only thing that distinguishes it from deterrence) which is that it involves the exercise of state power in such a way as to inhibit or disrupt behaviour that is morally valuable and should be protected.

This chapter cannot provide a full defence of a new theory of chill. However, it does suggest some ways in which the concept could be refined in order to better describe and capture the impact of police surveillance of protest movements. Specifically, recognizing that chilling effects occur at the level of the organization and not just the individual; that they can include a range of distorting and disruptive attitudinal and behavioural responses on the part of both observers and targets, and not just omissions or avoidances; and that, when targeted at protest movements, they always exert an inhibiting or disruptive effect on the exercise of political liberties. Adapted in these ways, the notion of chill could constitute an important conceptual tool in current debates about the surveillance of protest movements and beyond.[20] Protest and civil disobedience are a fundamental aspect of both normal and emergency politics in a democracy, as the public turn to activism in crises from climate change to the Covid-19 pandemic have illustrated. This chapter has argued that police surveillance exerts a chilling effect that is deleterious to legitimate protest movements and, as such, to democracy itself.

# References

Aston, V. 2017. State surveillance of protest and the rights to privacy and freedom of assembly: A comparison of judicial and protester perspectives. *European Journal of Law and Technology* 8 (1): 1–19.

APPG 'All Party Parliamentary Group on Democracy and the Constitution'. 2021. Police Power and the Right to Peaceful Protest. Institute for Constitutional and Democratic Research. At: https://www.icdr.co.uk/bristol-clapham-inquiry-home

Baker, D., S. Bronitt, and P. Stenning. 2017. 'Policing Protest, Security and Freedom: The 2014 G20 Experience'. *Police Practice and Research* 18 (5): 425–48.

---

[20] Is there a risk that the analysis here could be inverted to construct an argument in *favour* of overt and covert police surveillance of illegitimate and illegal protest movements, and indeed organized crime and terrorist groups? Unlike environmental movements, the mobilization of such groups is itself a source of threat to civil liberties and human rights, so there is little to lose by deterring or disrupting their activities. But while this line of argument is not unreasonable, and it is worth exploring these possibilities further, the conclusions are not foregone: there is some evidence suggesting that surveillance of organized crime groups can be self-defeating. For example, an in-depth account of the undercover infiltration of drugs markets found that police action drives them further underground and makes their leaders more dangerous and violent, as they seek to root out and punish suspected informants who are often the most vulnerable individuals at the margins of the organizations Woods 2017).

Bayley, D. H. 1985. *Patterns of Policing: A Comparative International Analysis*. Rutgers University Press.

BBC. 2021. 'Four Met Police officers injured in anti-vaccine protest'. 3rd Sept. 2021. At: https://www.bbc.co.uk/news/uk-england-london-58440700

Brownlee, K. 2012. *Conscience and Conviction: The Case for Civil Disobedience*. Oxford University Press.

Brownlee, K. 2012a. *Conscience and Conviction: The Case for Civil Disobedience*. Oxford University Press.

Bugden D. 2020. Does Climate Protest Work? Partisanship, Protest, and Sentiment Pools. *Socius*. 6, 1–13.

Burke, E., C. C. Collins, L. Bergeron et al. 2020. 'Teen Activism Leads to Local Laws Banning Single-Use Plastics: A Two-Year Experiential Learning Journey'. *Sustain Earth* 3: 15.

Casciani, D. 2021. 'Extinction Rebellion: Judge demands review of protester convictions'. BBC News, 4 August. At: https://www.bbc.co.uk/news/uk-58092234.

Catt vs The United Kingdom. 2019. European Court of Human Rights, Strasbourg (Application no. 43514/15), 24 April.

Dodd, V. and J. Grierson. 2020. The Guardian https://www.theguardian.com/uk-news/2020/jan/10/xr-extinction-rebellion-listed-extremist-ideology-police-prevent-scheme-guidance

Evans, R. and P. Lewis. 2012. 'Call for police links to animal rights firebombing to be investigated'. *The Guardian*, 13 Jun 2012. https://www.theguardian.com/uk/2012/jun/13/police

Evans, R. and P. Lewis. 2013. 'Police "Smear" Campaign Targeted Stephen Lawrence's Friends and Family'. *The Guardian*, 24 June 2013. https://www.theguardian.com/uk/2013/jun/23/stephen-lawrence-undercover-police-smears

First Witness Statement of HN301 to the Undercover Policing Inquiry. 2019. Ref.MPS-0742600. 25 October. At: https://www.ucpi.org.uk/publications/first-witness-statement-of-hn301/

Fisher, D. and S. Nasrin. 2020. Climate Activism and Its Effects. Wiley Interdisciplinary Reviews, Climate Change. 2021;12 1–11.

Gilmore, J., W. Jackson, H. Monk, and D. Short. 2020. Policing the UK's anti-fracking movement: facilitating peaceful protest or facilitating the industry? *Peace, Human Rights, Governance* 4 (3).

Glomsrød, S. and T. Wei. 2018. Business as unusual: The implications of fossil divestment and green bonds for financial flows, economic growth and energy market. *Energy for Sustainable Development*, 44, 1–10.

Haggerty, K. and M. Samatas. 2020. *Surveillance and Democracy*. Routledge.

HMICFRS 'Her Majesty's Inspectorate of Constabulary, Fire and Rescue Services' 2021. Getting the balance right? An inspection of how effectively the police deal with protests. At: https://www.justiceinspectorates.gov.uk/hmicfrs/publications/getting-the-balance-right-an-inspection-of-how-effectively-the-police-deal-with-protests/

Home Office. Police, Crime, Sentencing and Courts Bill 2021. UK Government. At: https://publications.parliament.uk/pa/bills/cbill/58-01/0268/200268.pdf

Kendrick, L. 2013. 'Speech, Intent, and the Chilling Effect' (2013) 54(5) William and Mary Law Review 1633.

Kyllönen, S. 2014. 'Civil Disobedience, Climate Protests and a Rawlsian Argument for "Atmospheric" Fairness'. *Environmental Values* 23 (5): 593–613.

Lubbers E. 2012. *Secret Manoevres in the Dark: Corporate and Police Spying on Activists*. Plutopress.

Mengesha v Commissioner of Police of the Metropolis [2013] EWHC 1695 (Admin) (18 June 2013) At: http://www.bailii.org/ew/cases/EWHC/Admin/2013/1695.html

Muñoz, J., S. Olzak, and S. A. Soule. 2018. Going green: Environmental protest, policy, and CO2 emissions in U.S. states, 1990–2007. *Sociological Forum*, 33 (2): 403–21

NPCC 'National Police Chiefs' Council'. 2022. Protest Operational Advice Document.

Opening Submissions on Behalf of Core Participants Represented By Hodge Jones & Allen, Bhatt Murphy and Bindmans Solicitors. https://www.ucpi.org.uk/wp-content/uploads/2020/11/20201026-Opening_Statement_CPs_represented-by_HJA_BM_Bindmans-MRQC.pdf

OSUPI 1. 'Opening statement to the Undercover Policing Inquiry on behalf of: Lois Austin Richard Chessum "Mary" Dave Nellist Hannah Sell Youth against Racism in Europe'. 20 October 2020. https://www.ucpi.org.uk/wp-content/uploads/2020/11/20201022-AMENDED_Opening_Statement-CPs_represented_by_PILC.pdf

Pech, L. 2021. 'The Concept of Chilling Effect: Its Untapped Potential to Better Protect Democracy, the Rule of Law, and Fundamental Rights in the EU'. Open Society European Policy Institute Report. Open Society Foundations.

PEN America. 201. 'Global Chilling: The Impact of Mass Surveillance on International Writers'. https://pen.org/research-resources/global-chilling/

Penney, J. 2016. 'Chilling Effects: Online Surveillance and Wikipedia Use'. *Berkeley Technology Law Journal* 31 (1): 117–82.

Penney, J. 2022. 'Understanding Chilling Effects'. 106 *Minnesota Law Review* Logical Forum 33 (2): 403–21.

Rawls, J. 1999. A Theory of Justice. Harvard University Press.

Rosane, O. 2019. '7.6 Million Join Week of Global Climate Strikes'. *EcoWatch*, 30 September 30. https://www.ecowatch.com/global-climate-strikes-week-2640790405.html

Saunders, C. and Price, S. 2009. One person's EU-topia, another's hell: Climate Camp as a heterotopia. Environmental Politics, 18:1, 117–122.

Schauer, F. 1978. 'Fear, Risk and the First Amendment: Unraveling the Chilling Effect'. *B.U. L. Rev.* 58: 685–732.

Schlembach, R. 2018. 'Undercover Policing and the Spectre of "Domestic Extremism": The Covert Surveillance of Environmental Activism in Britain'. *Social Movement Studies* 17 (5): 1.

Slaven, M. and J. Heydon. 2020. 'Crisis, Deliberation, and Extinction Rebellion'. *Critical Studies on Security* 8 (1): 59–62.

Starr, A. and others. 2008. 'The Impacts of State Surveillance on Political Assembly and Association: A Socio-Legal Analysis'. *Qualitative Sociology* 31 (3): 251.

Stoycheff, E. Burgess, S., and Martucci, M. 2020. 'Online Censorship and Digital Surveillance: The Relationship between Suppression Technologies and Democratization across Countries'. *Information, Communication & Society* 23 (4): 474–90.

Tucker, D. Interviewed by Cara McGoogan for Episode 7 'Inquiry, part II' of the Telegraph Newspaper podcast 'Bed of Lies', at minute 23–4.

Woods, N. 2017. *Good Cop, Bad War*. Ebury Press. Penguin.

# 9

# The Dynamics of Public Health Ethics

## Covid-19 and Surveillance as *Justifiable but Abnormal*

*Adam Henschke*

The issue that this paper is looking at is this—that what is permissible or even obligatory under public health emergencies ought to be treated as an exceptionalism. That is, while certain policies and practices might be permitted in response to the Covid-19 pandemic, we need to ensure not only that such policies are reversed once the Covid-19 emergency has receded but also that the social norms around particular practices and policies return to pre-Covid-19 states. The concern is that certain public health ethics principles that permit particular surveillance policies in emergency situations will become standardized social practices persisting after Covid-19. Underneath this claim is a recognition that public health ethics is not only pluralistic but dynamic. What is ethically justifiable changes given the context, and we need to recognize that this dynamic runs in two ways—not only do public health emergencies justify exceptional practices, but on a dynamic view, public health emergencies also end, and as such, so too do the exceptional justifications that arise in such emergencies.

The Covid-19 emergency has potentially driven a broader acceptance of public health ethics, and this could produce benefits, such as an increase in solidarity and awareness of the importance of public health. However, certain principles of public health ethics have potential negative consequences if they become normalized for situations beyond this emergency. By that I mean that what is ethically permissible or even obligatory during the legitimate public health emergency of Covid-19 may not be permissible in non-emergencies. We need to be careful with what we permit during the emergency and ensure that there are reversals on the permissions granted during the emergency. Given this, I argue that the surveillance policies and technologies introduced during the Covid-19 pandemic ought to be considered as *justifiable but abnormal*. As I will show, this categorization is particularly important for less immediately invasive policies like technologically enabled surveillance than other extreme measures like forced quarantine, forced vaccination, and the like. The point is that once the emergency ceases, we should not only scale back surveillance but need to attend to restoring social norms that

Adam Henschke, *The Dynamics of Public Health Ethics: Covid-19 and Surveillance as* Justifiable but Abnormal In: *The Ethics of Surveillance in Times of Emergency*. Edited by: Kevin Macnish and Adam Henschke, Oxford University Press.
© Oxford University Press 2023. DOI: 10.1093/oso/9780192864918.003.0010

existed before the emergency. While policy making during the emergency justifiably took its the lead from public health and was informed by public health ethics, and this policy making needed to be rapid, the moral hazard is that the surveillance practises that were necessary during the emergency remain, and that such pervasive surveillance is normalized.

## Covid-19 Driving New Surveillance Practices

During the Covid-19 pandemic, the globe was faced with a legitimate public health emergency. Many millions of people's lives were at risk, and extraordinary measures were taken to limit its spread and prevent massive direct and indirect deaths. Large-scale national policies that were unthinkable prior to 2020 became the norm as the pandemic continued. Emergency situations require extraordinary responses.[1] In the early stages of the pandemic, many countries activated biosecurity and emergency laws that gave governments extraordinary powers over people and institutions (Vinjamuri 2020; Karp 2020; Al Jazeera News And Agencies 2020). In the context of a global health emergency, extraordinary ethical justifications shifted to meet the emerging reality of the situation (Chotiner 2020; Grunau 2020). As part of the response, a number of countries and regions introduced surveillance practices that would normally have been illegal, so socially contentious as to be impermissible or drawn out through a long-winded public consultation.

The start of the pandemic saw a raft of abnormal practices rapidly introduce to deal with the emergency. Israel, for instance activated a set of technologies that allowed for surveillance of individuals through their mobile phones (Mitnick 2020; Estrin 2020; Halbfinger, Kershner, and Bergman 2020). This technology was an adaptation of existing counter-terrorism technologies and policies. These technologies gave their domestic security agency the Shin Bet the capacity to monitor the location and movement of potentially infectious individuals through their mobile phones, and to use meta-data to engage in contact tracing, establishing an awareness of the networks of infection and transmission (Cahane 2020). Thus, on this, not only was the privacy of the potentially infectious individuals who have been overridden, but so too was the privacy of those individuals they might have had some contact with. In this example, the need for comprehensive pandemic surveillance was deemed to be justified in order to better understand transmission and identify potential risks.

South Korea was initially extremely effective in its control of the spread and impact of the outbreak, at least in the early stages of the global outbreak (Bicker

---

[1] For more on this notion of 'emergency ethics', see (Viens and Selgelid 2012).

2020; Heejin Kee, Sohee Kim, and Claire Che 2020). One of the measures that they introduced was an expansion of surveillance technologies such that not only did the state health and security officials have access to data on the location and movements of potentially infectious individuals, but they also made this information publicly accessible. On this, the public was given access to information about the location and movements of potentially infectious individuals (Hyung Eun Kim 2020; Min Joo Kim and Denyer 2020). While it is those who were described by this technology had their identity protected (Hyung Eun Kim 2020) as privacy advocates have argued, with comprehensive surveillance technologies, anonymity is relatively easily reversed through the aggregation of multiple data sets (Henschke 2017; Solove 2008, 2004).[2] The rights of individuals to maintain the privacy of health relevant information and prevent that information from going public were deemed to be overridden by the public health emergency.

Spain was hit very hard by Covid-19 in its early stages (Sullivan et al. 2020). As the scale of the crisis expanded, Spain instituted a range of significant policies to enforce local lockdowns and physical distancing (BBC 2020). Drone technologies were used in Madrid to identify if there were groups of people in public in contravention of the orders for public shutdowns (Doffman 2020). Interestingly, these drones were also used to broadcast to these people that they were in contravention of the relevant lockdowns and, should people persist in ignoring the lockdowns, they would be individually identified by the police and either fined or imprisoned (Doffman 2020). Similarly, in the United Arab Emirates, drones were used to spray down public areas in an effort to decontaminate public areas (Belleza 2020).

While it is speculation, I suggest that as much as these efforts were sincere and evidence-based policies, the public displays were also an effort on behalf of governments to show their local populations that things were being done to stem the rates of infection. Moreover, they were motivated in part to show to people that their governments were actually able to do something (see Macnish in this volume). This goes to the idea of the theatre of security, where governments not only need to respond to particular threats, but citizens need to be assured that the government is still there and is doing something—'Cybersecurity writer and practitioner Bruce Schneier coined the term "security theatre' to describe and criticize security countermeasures that 'provide the feeling of security instead of

---

[2] I note here that others like Kevin Macnish offer a different analysis, that privacy is not synonymous with information control. On his view, '[s]eizing control of another's information is therefore harmful, even though it may not entail a violation of privacy' (Macnish 2018: 418). While I do not share this view, nothing in this paper stands or falls on how narrow or broad one's definition of privacy is. As Macnish notes, having others control your information can still be ethically problematic.

the reality' (Persad 2016: 588). As Govind Persad noted, there is a logic in extending the notion of security theatre to 'health theatre' (Persad 2016). Note that I do not think that the theatre of security or health are inherently problematic. Especially in times of significant public anxiety like that of the Covid-19 pandemic, people do need to observe and know that their governments are functioning and doing things. Of course, there are still significant ethical concerns with the theatre of security, not the least of which being the use of fear and anxiety to make ethically problematic policies and decisions seem acceptable. My reason for bringing it up is what role public displays of contravention of standard norms play in shifting what is publicly acceptable policy.

The overall point of this section is to show that in extreme situations like those faced by the globe in the initial phases of the Covid-19 pandemic, what would normally be prohibited becomes normal, even obligatory. Widespread state surveillance of innocent individuals, the publicizing of people's health status, the use of drones as public control and assurance devices, these are all phenomena that were only permitted given the emergency being faced. And, what is relevant for this paper, is that not only were these measures (and many others) deemed justifiable, it seemed that many people in countries as diverse as Israel, South Korea, Spain, and the United Arab Emirates were happy to assent to such measures.

## Public Health Ethics Normalizing New Surveillance

This is all to say that during the Covid-19 pandemic, not only did public health become arguably the most pressing global issue, but also that 'public health ethics' became a significantly more mainstream frame for discussing how to structure and order societies. By public health ethics I mean the cluster of ethical concerns which not only focus on ethical issues of public health but also argue or imply that the ethics of public health are important and in situations of a public health emergency, such public considerations change our ethical calculus. This includes discussion of issues such as:

> the measures required for the protection of public health may include surveillance; mandatory vaccination, testing or treatment; and/or social distancing measures such as isolation and quarantine. Though measures like these may sometimes promote the greater good of society in the way of public health or utility (i.e., aggregate well- being), they each conflict with widely acknowledged basic human rights and liberties. Surveillance conflicts with (the right to) privacy; mandatory vaccination, testing and treatment conflict with (the right to) informed consent to medical intervention; and coercive social distancing measures conflict with (the right to) freedom of movement.   (Selgelid 2009: 196)

Part of the challenge of ethics and infectious diseases are that '[b]ecause (in most cases) infectious diseases are spread from person to person, innocent individuals can present a threat to other innocent individuals ... Restrictions of liberty and incursions of privacy and confidentiality may be necessary to promote the public good' (Selgelid et al. 2009: 150). As Michael Selenide astutely observed in 2010, 'public health measures—such as contact tracing, the notification of third parties, and the reporting of the health status of individuals to authorities— can interfere with the right to privacy' (Selgelid 2010, 430). On Selgelid's analysis, '[i]f a disastrous epidemic would result from the maximal protection of individual rights and liberties, then individual rights and liberties must be compromised' (Selgelid 2010: 435). Importantly, Selgelid is not saying that just any public health situations warrant such abrogation of individual liberties, this can only be justified in situations of a disastrous epidemic. '[A]n extreme measure such as quarantine should not be imposed unless the consequences of failing to do so would be great. It would be wrong to think that rights violations and the imposition of harms on individuals are justified whenever this would lead to a net pay-off for society as a whole' (Selgelid 2010: 435). Such a forfeiture of individual rights is only that—they are forfeited for the short term and individuals still maintain other legal and moral rights. Moreover, as Selgelid argues, the conditions of quarantine must be minimally burdensome and the individuals subject to quarantine might be owed compensation as a result of their quarantine (Selgelid 2010: 436).

The point here is that in public health ethics, we find a basis for why significant interference with individual liberty can potentially be justified, but that other values must also be factored into our analysis and treatment of those individuals. On this public health ethics analysis, the situation with at the start of Covid-19 was one where an increasingly disastrous epidemic was facing the globe, and extreme measures were ethically justifiable. Thus, widespread use of surveillance technologies was considered to be ethically justifiable. In addition, the general application of public health ethics was also seen by many as appropriate.

As noted by Selgelid, in situations of public health emergencies, governments and societies more generally may need to take extreme measures to limit infections and the spread of the disease. During the Covid-19 pandemic, these measures included practices like forced quarantine, the closing of national even state or county borders, the shut-down of many businesses and public areas and increasingly aggressive laws to punish those who broke such directives. In China there were even reports of the doors of people's homes being welded shut in efforts to contain people inside (Guangcheng 2020). Such policies were obviously significant curtailments in the basic right or freedom to free movement or assembly, something that many nations and societies take for granted. Such laws contravene very basic rights of bodily autonomy. The start of the Covid-19 pandemic saw instantiations of the trade-offs between public health and individual liberties, with public health often outweighing individual liberties.

My interest, however, is on the widespread introduction of new permissions for surveillance policies and technologies. The reason is that the policies that resulted in the deprivation of free movement or bodily autonomy are not only extreme but easy to observe. Moreover, they were the first of the policies to be rescinded, in no small part because people rightfully resent having these rights curtailed and want things to return to normal—widespread and ongoing protests about lockdowns and vaccine mandates have continued and in some places picked up as the pandemic has dragged on. Almost two years after the pandemic began, Ottawa was besieged by protesters opposed to vaccine mandates (*BBC News* 2022). In contrast, many of the surveillance practices are largely invisible and/or seemingly ethically unproblematic or innocuous.[3] By habit, many of us carry our phones on us and likely saw no real difference if those phones were tracking us. Likewise, for many of us, we are increasingly becoming familiar with drones appearing in public places. They are no longer a shocking new technology but becoming part of the background of modern life. These surveillance practices and technologies were much more easily part of normal life under Covid-19 than the other more extreme policies.

The main points here are that, on a public health ethics analysis, new policies like increased surveillance were not only justified by a public health emergency, but also that surveillance practices were accepted as a necessary part of the need to respond to the pandemic. At the start of the Covid-19 pandemic, emergency measures were justified by a public health ethics that normalized new and more pervasive surveillance. I mean normalized here in two senses—one is in the ethical sense, and one is in the social sense. 'Moral norms are *moral judgments*. Social norms are clusters of normative attitudes of some other kinds,—*social judgments* we might say' (emphases original; Brennan et al. 2013: 58). The Covid-19 pandemic saw that the public health emergency justified new surveillance practices. As with many people, I think that the Covid-19 pandemic was a legitimate public health emergency that warranted extraordinary responses. Like quarantine and forced physical distancing, the surveillance was ethically justifiable.[4] I also mean 'normalized' in the broader sense of a social norm. Here I mean something more like 'the purely *statistical* sense of "norm" as simply noting what is common or habitual' (emphasis original; Brennan et al. 2013: 2). Here, what is

---

[3] I have written in detail elsewhere how the gathering and use of innocuous information can in fact be ethically problematic (Henschke 2017).

[4] One point here is that I do not want to say that every instance of increased surveillance or every policy around surveillance was ethically justified. There were likely many instances where such surveillance was ethically problematic. My point is more general, that on the public health ethics frame, given the global emergency, that such surveillance and other measures were potentially ethically justifiable (see Macnish, chapter 12 in this volume).

common becomes normalized, becomes the norm. In the Covid-19 pandemic, surveillance and other emergency measures became socially normalized. They became common. This was in part because people accepted them as a descriptive fact about their world at the time. And in part, because people accepted them, they became common. There is, I suggest a necessary logical connection between the ethical norms—we need to permit these new policies to limit the impact of the pandemic—with the social norms—because these policies are necessary, we simply need to let them become standardized.[5] Again, I suggest that this is definitely the case with many of the surveillance policies and technologies. Because people saw, and largely agreed with, the need for these policies and technologies, they allowed them to become common, the new surveillance policies and technologies became normal.

## Public Health Ethics as Dynamic

So far, the focus in the chapter has been on the initiating features of emergency measures. My point in this section is draw out a feature of public health ethics as being dynamic. By that I mean that not only must we consider different factors when considering what is justifiable in events like the Covid-19 pandemic than in normal conditions, but also that those considerations shift as the reality shifts. I start with an endorsement of the ethically pluralistic nature of public health emergences. As Selgelid has argued at length (Selgelid 2008, 2009, 2010, 2012; Selgelid et al. 2009, Selgelid and Enemark 2008), when considering public health generally, and particularly when considering issues like pandemics, a singular or monistic ethics simply does not work. Our deliberations and policy development cannot just consider one value or ethical system like personal freedom, the overall utility of a given policy and we cannot overlook issues of equality and fairness.

The pluralism here draws from two related aspects. First, it seeks to recognize that ethics generally is an open question. '[N]o amount of philosophical argument can lead to a definitive victory of one account of value over the rest. Moral reflection is the effort to bring different dimensions of value to bear on specific occasions of judgment and to determine how they are best balanced or ordered, given the facts of the case' (Galston 2002: 6). This pluralism is a descriptive fact of life, at least in liberally minded societies, where we claim to hold 'the idea that there are many viable conceptions of the good life that neither represent different

---

[5] On the larger metaethical issue of the relations between ethics and society, I do not think much of that is relevant for this paper. By that I mean, is ethics the result of individual reason/rationality, or something more like the social intuitionist model advocated by Jonathan Haidt (Haidt 2012, 2001). Despite the importance of these debates, I do not think that what I say in this paper stands or falls on which position one takes.

versions of some single, homogenous good, nor fall into any discernible hierarchy' (Larmore 1987: 23). Expanding beyond a view that just looks at 'the good life', 'a complete account will need to appeal to several foundational theories, each one of which is able to explain the basis of *some* of the normative factors, but no one of which explains all of them' (Kagan 1998: 294–5; emphasis original). For instance, a utilitarian will likely differ from a libertarian in how a solution for moral disagreements ought to be decided.

> The problem with utilitarianism and libertarianism is that they each place extreme, and arguably implausible, weight on the values they emphasize. Utilitarianism holds that utility takes absolute priority—and that liberties must be compromised whenever liberty restriction is required to maximally promote utility overall (i.e., over the long run, all things considered). Libertarianism, on the other hand, calls for the opposite: (negative) liberty takes priority and must not be infringed for the sake of utility.   (Selgelid 2009: 196)

Thus, there are a range of different answers that one look to tell us what we ought to do generally, and in public health emergencies.[6]

Second, following Selgelid again, *each* of these nominated values are important. On this form of pluralism, it is not simply that liberty, utility, and justice may offer different explanations and justifications for a given decision or policy, it is also that *all* of these must play a role in decision making and good policy formation. We cannot simply say that utility reigns supreme in pandemic situations, even if individuals are to lose some rights or liberties, they do not lose them all. Even if they are in lockdown, for instance, individuals retain the right for basic recognition respect.[7] Moreover, the procedural and resource aspects of justice must be taken into account—if people are to suffer the deprivation of their liberties, they are owed explanations and may be owed compensation for those deprivations (Selgelid 2010). I consider that such a pluralistic approach, where there may be differing views, can be founded in a narrow set of values like basic recognition, the duty to reduce suffering and a commitment to fairness, apply to surveillance policies too. As I have argued at length, when living in an age of surveillance, while certain policies and technologies might be ethically justified, such surveillance must be justified by reference to these values (Henschke 2017).

Having spelled out that I think pluralism obtains in situations like Covid-19, where multiple ethical values must be considered for decision making, the main

---

[6] I note here that on such a form of pluralism, it is deliberately distinct from an ethical relativism where 'anything goes'. Though it is an open question what ethical system is or are the correct one(s), there are a narrow range of values that count as authoritative to justify particular actions or decisions.

[7] I refer here to Stephen Darwall's work which suggests a distinction between recognition and appraisal respect (Darwall 1977). I talk in more detail about recognition respect and surveillance in *Ethics in an Age of Surveillance* (Henschke 2017: 208–15).

point I wish to make is that such considerations are not just pluralistic but *dynamic*. Many of the policies that shifted our ethical calculus were only justified given the extreme threat that the globe faced. Certain of these policies, for instance those that permitted widespread surveillance on collective public health grounds, would not be justifiable in normal circumstances. This, I think, is obvious and uncontroversial when considering policies like forced quarantine and the shutting down of public spaces. We may accept that in the extraordinary circumstances like a global pandemic, particular policies are both justifiable and become accepted, but these policies are *abnormal*. It is only because of the real and significant threat faced around the globe that such policies become permissible.

Further, while it may be obvious certain policies are short lived, it is important to highlight that the ethical permissions granted by the emergency are limited to the emergency—the policies and particular applications of the technologies only become permissible because of the threat. Under normal circumstances, the policies and technologies would not be justified or accepted. That is, certain of the public health ethics justifications only become operational due to the type and magnitude of the threat being faced. The point here is that not only do they become justifiable when the conditions of the threat arise, but that the justifications recede as the threat recedes. While we find justifications and acceptance for these policies and technologies, as soon as the threat is properly dealt with, these policies and technologies lose their justifications and need to be reversed. That is, this is a dynamic space.

What I would suggest here is that the policies and technologies permitted during the Covid-19 pandemic be classified as *justifiable but abnormal*. Such classifications are important as they signal that, while some policy or practice is justified, we need to see it as abnormal, and need to return to a pre-emergency norm once the threat ceases. A similar argument exists in relation to the potential justifiability of torture (Henschke 2016). In particular circumstances, such as a ticking time bomb where the security forces reliably know that torturing a specific terrorist would save thousands of lives, what is normally impermissible becomes potentially justifiable. However, such situations need to be seen as necessary *but still evil*. While the torture might be justified, given a significant number of caveats and constraints, in order to save thousands of lives, it is still an evil, something that is normally ethically impermissible. By describing such situations as necessary *but still evil*, rather than a lesser evil, we preserve the norm that torture is an ethically impermissible action. Likewise, in situations like that faced in global pandemics, we need to see particular policies as *justifiable but abnormal*.

The point of this classification, *justifiable but abnormal*, is to capture and reinforce the notion that certain of our policies are outside the social norm. While we might find that they could be ethically justified, we need to actively recognize that they are undesirable to maintain as social norms beyond the time that the policies lose their ethical justifiability. The driving concern is that norms are sticky—their slowness to change—is of course a familiar feature of norms' (Brennan et al. 2013: 108). Once a social norm is established, it takes effort to change that norm. Emergencies like the Covid-19 pandemic brought about a rapid change to social norms, and the concern is that the new social norms remain, 'stick around' after the emergency has passed. By drawing attention to the recognition that policies and technologies like pandemic surveillance are abnormal, we have a better chance of minimizing that stickiness.

This ties together two strands of the paper so far. First, the recognition of a difference between ethical norms and social norms. What is ethically justifiable ought to still be considered socially abnormal, something that is only justified in special circumstances. Second, it relies on the recognition that these public health ethics are dynamic. Not only do they only become activated in special circumstances, but we want things to return to the pre-emergency situation when they can. This is especially important for policies relating to, and technologies of, surveillance. While we can easily recognize that forced quarantine etc., are abnormal policies and that a return to normal is desirable, I suggest that it easier to treat changes to surveillance policies and technologies as the new normal. They need to be considered *justifiable but abnormal*.

As a final point in this section, I note that a number of the policies might feasibly remain justified after the threat recedes. For instance, on Selgelid's account, one of the main things that public health ethics requires is a far greater investment into healthcare in low-income countries (Selgelid 2008, 2010; Selgelid and Enemark 2008) and in so called 'tropical diseases'. Similarly, we saw many nations institute a range of healthcare and social welfare programmes to help protect low income and vulnerable members of their populations. On this, I would suggest that such policies ought to remain, but are justified differently to the ethical justifications that arose during the pandemic. That is, while those policies were brought in because of the pandemic, there are a range of lo general ethical arguments as to why such policies ought to remain, that are not linked to the threat of Covid-19. See, for instance (Daniels 2008; Resnik 2004; Schuklenk and Ashcroft 2000; Scott 2008; Selgelid 2008, 2009; Selgelid and Enemark 2008; Pogge 2001, 2005, 2008). My point here is that the specific justifications that are active during the pandemic do fall away, but there may be more general ethical justifications that hold significant weight for particular policies. On the dynamic approach, these policies would lose the specific pandemic justifications, but this does not mean they are no longer justifiable.

## Ensuring That Surveillance Remains Abnormal

I have so far argued that Covid-19 brought in a raft of surveillance policies and technologies that would have been largely impermissible and unacceptable in normal circumstances. I next argued that this is because, like a number of policies, in such a public health emergency, these policies and technologies were both justifiable and largely acceptable. I then suggested that we need to see public health ethics, and the policies and technologies of surveillance, as dynamic, that not only do certain of the public health ethics justifications only become operationalized in extreme circumstances, but also that they ought to be reversed. We need to ensure that certain of our social norms return to pre-pandemic normality. In this section I argue why we want to revert the social norms around surveillance to pre-pandemic standards and offer some suggestions about how we can check if this is happening.

In terms of the surveillance, one concern is function creep. Surveillance technologies originally used for one purpose can be used for other purposes. Consider the Amazon Ring, a camera mounted at the front door of people's homes that can be remotely accessed to see who is at the door. The Ring technology was subsequently used in the US by a number of different policing agencies to gather information on people on the public street (Harwell 2019). The point here is that, like mobile phones, the multipurposing of these surveillance technologies can allow for a range of new uses. Moreover, what is particularly relevant is that this function creep can occur invisibly, without the necessary knowledge of the device's primary user or owner. Here, a key element of function creep is the capacity to shift the device's use remotely. The changes in use and function can potentially occur by the decision and actions of people remote from the primary user and owner of the device.

Parallel with the function creep is what we might call 'user creep': Not only can the use change remotely, but the range of *users* can also change. One of the significant capacities of digital technologies is that the information they produce can be used and reused by individuals at a remove from the initial user or owner. First, '[I]nformation doesn't wear out. It [can] be endlessly recycled [and] repackaged' (Drahos and Braithwaite 2002: 58–9). Many different people can use this information. Second, with the interconnectedness of many of our devices, that information can be communicated and shared instantaneously. Third, this sharing of information happens in a way in which those who access and use the information are potentially hidden from the original sources of the information.[8] Put these three elements together and you have the potential for a whole range of new users to access and apply surveillance information in ways at a remove from the original purpose and the original user of that information. The Covid-19 pandemic was a driver of both function creep and user creep.

---

[8] In his 2004 book *The Digital Person*, Daniel Solove convincingly argued that we ought to see information technologies like surveillance technologies as 'Kafkaesque' in that the users of this information and their motives can easily be hidden from the sources and targets of such surveillance (Solove 2004: 27–55).

This leads us to ask why we should be worried about these new uses and users of surveillance technologies? I have argued elsewhere that we need global pandemic surveillance networks (Henschke 2017: 253). Such a capacity is needed in our globally connected world, as it is only a matter of time until the next pandemic outbreak, a point strongly made by Laurie Garret from the mid-1990s (Garrett 1996, 2001). On the other hand, what is so wrong or ethically problematic about such surveillance? We live our lives online, posting the most intimate details of our personal lives publicly. Privacy, it is often said, is dead, no longer a social norm (Henschke 2017: 28–55). So, on the one hand we have reasons to think that pandemic surveillance is a good thing, and on the other hand, we might be sceptical about privacy arguments against surveillance.

I do not have the space to detail arguments against widespread surveillance and in favour of privacy here. Daniel Solove (2004, 2008); Jeroen van den Hoven (van den Hoven 2007, 2008; van den Hoven and Vermaas 2007); Elliot Cohen (2010); Helen Nissenbaum (2009); and Adam Henschke (Robbins and Henschke 2017; Henschke 2017) have presented different forms of these arguments. Instead, I will simply stipulate that the two main reasons are first that privacy is a fundamentally and/or instrumentally valuable thing, necessary for personal development, intimate relationships, and social cohesion (Koops et al. 2016). Second, that privacy is often a useful protection against government overreach (Henschke 2020). As was documented during the Covid-19 pandemic, a number of governments with authoritarian tendencies used the Covid-19 pandemic as a way of extending their power and decreasing the power of their citizens (Gebrekidan 2020). Moreover, when considering government surveillance, we face the potential of 'an "informational deficit", where the state's knowledge about its citizens substantially surpasses what the citizens know about the state. While there has always been some informational deficit between what a state does and what its citizens know, the worry here is that the new technologies provide so much more information about its people, without a corresponding increase in the citizens knowing about the state' (Robbins and Henschke 2017: 583). Not only does widespread surveillance degrade privacy rights, and offer the potential for abuse and misuse of power by the state and other institutions, it can significantly impact state–citizen relations. In short, while certain surveillance policies and technologies might be justifiable, we need to be very careful about how such policies and technologies are used and applied.

To close off, I offer some suggestions on how we ensure that the surveillance justified by public health ethics remains abnormal. The first step is to look closely at the 'moral mechanics' that justified the surveillance. We need to look closely at the ethical justifications offered in support of the new policies and technologies; what was justified, for how long, why, whose rights were violated, what were the costs and how were those costs distributed? In parallel, we need to see such public health ethics as a form of exceptionalism. On this, which four elements must be provided as part of the justification for the particular decision? An exceptionalism should first 'tell us what the exception is *to*. Second, it should tell us *what* is being excepted. Third, it should properly delimit the *scope* of the exceptions. Fourth, it should tell us *why* the exception is being made' (Emphases Original Allhoff 2012: 40). These four elements seek to treat the situation as justifiable but abnormal; they take seriously the pre-pandemic social norms and seek to preserve them.

The second step is to recognize that public health officials have a responsibility to make sure that the policies themselves are in fact justified. That is, did the surveillance policies and technologies actually help with containing and reducing the pandemic? While it is obvious to see how widespread surveillance might help in a pandemic in theory, we need to see if these theories actually helped in practice. This is the important distinction between a policy or technology being 'justifiable' and it being 'justified'. For instance, while surveillance of infected individuals might have been useful for tracking the spread of infections and contact tracing, is there any evidence to show that publicly communicating information about potentially infectious people was useful? Likewise, did the use of drones actually objectively help the situation or were they merely part of theatre of security? Sahar Latheef's entry in this collection explores these questions to suggest that a number of surveillance technologies were in fact of limited use. As such, these surveillance tools ought to be removed and we can be concerned about their use in the future.

Third, there was a responsibility on policy makers, to both listen to public health experts in crafting the new laws, as well as to make sure that the policies are written such that they are not simply reversible but will be reversed by default. This draws from the recognition that public health ethics are dynamic. Policymakers and relevant experts in health and security law need to be able to revisit those laws and to review them in order to see that they are in fact reversed if no ongoing justification remains.

Fourth, ethicists have a responsibility to make sure that the moral mechanics are right. It is not enough to simply say that these policies and technologies are justifiable, we need to ask were they in fact *justified*? If they were not, why weren't they justified, and what can be learnt from this so that we do not permit such repeats in the future? Further, like the responsibility on policy makers, ethicists need to review the laws and policies to make sure that those that have lost their justifications are in fact reversed. And where they have not been reversed, such policies need to be publicly criticized.

Finally, a range of public communicators have a responsibility to make sure that the abnormality of these policies is recognized and reinforced. As I have argued, we should not simply be concerned with the ethical norms that justified these policies and technologies, but we also need to attend to the social norms that shifted during the pandemic. Insofar as such social norms could be changed, we need to engage the public at large to see that these social norms are reversed.

To finish, this is why recognizing the dynamic nature of public health ethics generally, and describing these policies as *justifiable but abnormal* in particular, becomes so practically important. Surveillance policies and technologies have a way of more easily becoming normalized than other public health measures enacted during the Covid-19 pandemic. We must consider not only that public health ethics may need to return to the pre-pandemic conditions but that social norms around surveillance policies and technologies may remain after the justifications recede. If this is the case, we need to actively pursue public actions that will return these norms from their abnormal state.

# References

Al Jazeera News and Agencies. 2020. 'UK: Coronavirus Emergency Bill to Become Law in Days'. *Al Jazeera*, 26 March. Accessed 1 April. https://www.aljazeera.com/news/2020/03/uk-coronavirus-emergency-bill-law-days-200325175754049.html.

Allhoff, Fritz. 2012. *Terrorism, Ticking Time-Bombs, and Torture*. Chicago: The University of Chicago Press.

BBC. 2020. 'Coronavirus: Spain and France Announce Sweeping Restrictions'. *BBC*, 15 March. Accessed 1 April 2020. https://www.bbc.com/news/world-europe-51892477.

BBC News. 2022. 'Freedom Convoy: Ottawa Declares Emergency over Trucker Covid Rules Protests', 7 February 2022, sec. US & Canada. https://www.bbc.com/news/world-us-canada-60281088.

Belleza, Irish Eden. 2020. 'Coronavirus Prevention: Dubai Uses Drones to Sterilise Streets'. *Gulf News*, 28 March.

Bicker, Laura. 2020. 'Coronavirus in South Korea: How "Trace, Test and Treat" May Be Saving Lives'. *BBC*, 12 March. Accessed 1 April 2020. https://www.bbc.com/news/world-asia-51836898.

Brennan, Geoffrey, Lina Eriksson, Robert E. Goodin, and Nicholas Southwood. 2013. *Explaining Norms*. Oxford: Oxford University Press.

Cahane, Amir. 2020. 'The Israeli Emergency Regulations for Location Tracking Of Coronavirus Carriers'. *Lawfare*, 21 March. https://www.lawfareblog.com/israeli-emergency-regulations-location-tracking-coronavirus-carriers.

Chotiner, Isaac. 2020. 'The Medical Ethics of the Coronavirus Crisis'. *The New Yorker*, 11 March.

Cohen, Elliot D. 2010. *Mass Surveillance and State Control*: Palgrave Macmilllan.

Daniels, Norman. 2008. *Just Health: Meeting Health Needs Fairly*. 1st ed. Cambridge: Cambridge University Press.

Darwall, Stephen L. 1977. 'Two Kinds of Respect'. *Ethics* 88 (1): 36–49.

Doffman, Zak. 2020. 'Coronavirus Spy Drones Hit Europe: This Is How They're Now Used'. *Forbes*, 16 March. Accessed 1 April 2020. https://www.forbes.com/sites/zakdoffman/2020/03/16/coronavirus-spy-drones-hit-europe-police-surveillance-enforces-new-covid-19-lockdowns/.

Drahos, Peter and John Braithwaite. 2002. *Information Feudalism: Who Owns the Knowledge Economy?* London: Earthscan.

Estrin, Daniel. 2020. 'Israel Begins Tracking and Texting Those Possibly Exposed to the Coronavirus'. *NPR*, 19 March.

Galston, William. 2002. *Liberal Pluralism: The Implications of Value Pluralism for Political Theory and Practice.* Cambridge: Cambridge University Press.

Garrett, Laurie. 1996. *The Coming Plague*: Penguin Books.

Garrett, Laurie. 2001. *Betrayal of Trust*: Hyperion books.

Gebrekidan, Selam. 2020. 'For Autocrats, and Others, Coronavirus Is a Chance to Grab Even More Power'. *New York Times*, 30 March. Accessed 1 April 2020. https://www.nytimes.com/2020/03/30/world/europe/coronavirus-governments-power.html.

Grunau, Andrea. 2020. 'Coronavirus and Ethics: "Act So That Most People Survive"'. *Deutsche Welle*, 24 March. Accessed 1 April 2020. https://www.dw.com/en/coronavirus-and-ethics-act-so-that-most-people-survive/a-52895179.

Guangcheng, Chen. 2020. 'Warning: Chinese Authoritarianism Is Hazardous to Your Health'. *The Washington Post*, 7 February. Accessed 1 April 2020. https://www.washingtonpost.com/opinions/2020/02/06/warning-chinese-authoritarianism-is-hazardous-your-health/.

Haidt, Jonathan. 2001. 'The Emotional Dog and Its Rational Tail: A Social Intuitionist Approach to Moral Judgment'. *Psychological Review* 108 (4): 814–34.

Haidt, Jonathan. 2012. *The Righteous Mind: Why Good People Are Divided by Politics And Religion.* London: Penguin.

Halbfinger, David M., Isabel Kershner, and Ronen Bergman. 2020. 'To Track Coronavirus, Israel Moves to Tap Secret Trove of Cellphone Data'. *New York Times*, 16 March. Accessed 1 April 2020. https://www.nytimes.com/2020/03/16/world/middleeast/israel-coronavirus-cellphone-tracking.html.

Harwell, Drew. 2019. 'Doorbell-Camera Firm Ring Has Partnered with 400 Police Forces, Extending Surveillance Concerns'. *Washington Post*, 29 August. Accessed 1 April, 2020. https://www.washingtonpost.com/technology/2019/08/28/doorbell-camera-firm-ring-has-partnered-with-police-forces-extending-surveillance-reach/.

Heejin Kee, Sohee Kim, and Claire Che. 2020. 'Virus Testing Blitz Appears to Keep Korea Death Rate Low'. *Bloomberg Businessweek*, 5 March. Accessed 1 April 2020. https://www.bloomberg.com/news/articles/2020-03-04/south-korea-tests-hundreds-of-thousands-to-fight-virus-outbreak.

Henschke, Adam. 2016. 'Sliding Off Torture's Halo of Prohibition: Lessons on the Morality of Torture Post 9/11'. *Asia-Pacific Journal on Human Rights and the Law* 17: 227–39.

Henschke, Adam. 2017. *Ethics in an Age of Surveillance: Virtual Identities and Personal Information.* New York: Cambridge University Press.

Henschke, Adam. 2020. 'Privacy, The Internet of Things and State Surveillance: Handling Personal Information within an Inhuman System'. *Moral Philosophy and Politics* 7 (1): 123.

Hyung Eun Kim. 2020. 'Coronavirus Privacy: Are South Korea's Alerts Too Revealing?' *BBC*, 5 March. Accessed 1 April. https://www.bbc.com/news/world-asia-51733145.

Kagan, Shelly. 1998. *Normative Ethics, Dimensions of Philosophy.* Boulder: Westview Press.

Karp, Paul. 2020. 'Coronavirus: What Power Does the Australian Government Have Over You During Crisis?'. *The Guardian*, 3 March. Accessed 1 April 2020. https://www.theguardian.com/world/2020/mar/03/coronavirus-what-legal-power-does-the-australian-government-have-to-respond-to-the-threat.

Koops, Bert-Jaap, Bryce Clayton Newell, Tjerk Timan, Ivan Skorvanek, Tomislav Chokrevski, and Masa Galic. 2016. 'A Typology of Privacy'. *University of Pennsylvania Journal of International Law* 38: 483.

Larmore, Charles. 1987. *Patterns of Moral Complexity.* Cambridge: Cambridge University Press.

Macnish, Kevin. 2018. 'Government Surveillance and Why Defining Privacy Matters in a Post-Snowden World'. *Journal of Applied Philosophy* 35 (2): 417–32.

Min Joo Kim and Simon Denyer. 2020. 'A "Travel Log" of the Times in South Korea: Mapping the Movements of Coronavirus Carriers'. *The Washington Post*, 14 March. Accessed 1 April 2020. https://www.washingtonpost.com/world/asia_pacific/coronavirus-south-korea-tracking-apps/2020/03/13/2bed568e-5fac-11ea-ac50-18701e14e06d_story.html.

Mitnick, Joshua. 2020. 'Better Health Through Mass Surveillance? Israeli Authorities Want to Spy on People with the Coronavirus'. *Foreign Policy*, 16 March.

Nissenbaum, Helen. 2009. *Privacy in Context: Technology, Policy, and the Integrity of Social Life.* Stanford: Stanford Law Books.

Persad, Govind. 2016. 'Health Theater'. *Loyola University of Chicago Law Journal* 48: 585.

Pogge, Thomas. 2001. 'Priorities of Global Justice'. *Metaphilosophy* 32 (1&2): 6–24. doi: doi:10.1111/1467-9973.00172.

Pogge, Thomas. 2005. 'Human Rights and Global Health: A Research Program'. *Metaphilosophy* 36 (1/2): 182–209.

Pogge, Thomas. 2008. *World Poverty and Human Rights.* 2nd ed. Cambridge: Polity Press.

Resnik, David B. 2004. 'The Distribution of Biomedical Research Resources and International Justice'. *Developing World Bioethics* 4 (1): 42–57. doi: doi:10.1111/j.1471-8731.2004.00066.x.

Robbins, Scott and Adam Henschke. 2017. 'Designing for Democracy: Bulk Data and Authoritarianism'. *Surveillance And Society* 15 (3): 582–9.

Schuklenk, Udo and Richard Ashcroft. 2000. 'International Research Ethics'. *Bioethics* 14: 158–72.

Scott, Charity. 2008. 'Belief in a Just World: A Case Study in Public Health Ethics'. *Hastings Center Report* 38 (1): 16.

Selgelid, Michael J. 2008. 'Improving Global Health: Counting Reasons Why'. *Developing World Bioethics* 8 (2): 115–25.

Selgelid, Michael J. 2009. 'A Moderate Pluralist Approach to Public Health Policy and Ethics'. *Public Health Ethics* 2 (2): 195–205. doi: 10.1093/phe/php018.

Selgelid, Michael. 2010. 'Infectious Diseases'. In *A Companion To Bioethics*, edited by Helga Kuhse and Peter Singer, 430–40. Malden: Wiley-Blackwell.

Selgelid, Michael. 2012. 'The Value Of Security: A Moderate Pluralist Perspective'. In *Ethics and Security Aspects of Infectious Disease Control: Interdisciplinary Perspectives*, edited by Christian Enemark and Michael Selgelid. Farnham: Ashgate.

Selgelid, Michael J. and Christian Enemark. 2008. 'Infectious Diseases, Secuirty and Ethics: The Case of HIV/AIDS'. *Bioethics* 22 (9): 457–65.

Selgelid, Michael J., Angela R. McLean, Nimalan Arinaminpathy, and Julian Savulescu. 2009. 'Infectious Disease Ethics: Limiting Liberty in Contexts of Contagion'. *Bioethical Inquiry* 6: 149–52. doi: 10.1007/s11673-009-9166-1.

Solove, Daniel. 2004. *The Digital Person: Technology and Privacy in the Information Age*. New York: New York University Press.

Solove, Daniel. 2008. *Understanding Privacy*. Harvard: Harvard University Press.

Sullivan, Helen, Kevin Rawlinson, Alexandra Topping, and Damien Gayle. Accessed 1 April 2020. 'Spain Overtakes China as Second Worst-Hit Country by COVID-19—As It Happened'. *The Guardian*, 26 March. Accessed 1 April 2020. https://www.theguardian.com/australia-news/live/2020/mar/25/coronavirus-live-news-india-lockdown-italy-cases-restrictions-uk-us-outbreak-australia-china-hubei-latest-updates.

van den Hoven, Jeroen. 2007. 'Privacy and the Varieties of Informational Wrongdoing'. In *Computer Ethics*, edited by John Weckert, 317–30. Aldershot: Ashgate Publishing.

van den Hoven, Jeroen. 2008. 'Information Technology, Privacy and the Protection of Personal Data'. In *Information Technology And Moral Philosophy*, edited by Jeroen van den Hoven and John Weckert, 301–21. Cambridge: Cambridge University Press.

van den Hoven, Jeroen, and Pieter Vermaas. 2007. 'Nano-Technology and Privacy: On Continuous Surveillance Outside the Panopticon'. *Journal of Medicine and Philosophy* 32 (3): 283–97.

Viens, Adrian M. and Michael Selgelid, eds. 2012. *Emergency Ethics*. London: Palgrave.

Vinjamuri, Lesli. 2020. 'America's Coronavirus Response Is Shaped by Its Federal Structure'. *Chatham House*, 16 March. Accessed 1 April, 2020. https://www.chathamhouse.org/expert/comment/americas-coronavirus-response-shaped-its-federal-structure.

# PART III

# ETHICS BY DESIGN IN SURVEILLANCE PROGRAMMES

# 10

# Ethical Requirements for Digital Systems for Contact Tracing in Pandemics

## A Solution to the Contextual Limits of Ethical Guidelines

*Björn Lundgren*

## Introduction

After being officially discovered in China in December 2019, the virus SARS-CoV-2—which causes the disease Covid-19—has spread to most of the world's countries. At the time of writing, some treatments and many vaccines have become available, while others are still being tested and developed. Efforts to minimize the spread also include so-called 'digital tracking and tracing systems' ('DTTSs'), some of which are already available and in use (O'Neill et al. 2020). Henceforth, by 'DTTS', I broadly mean any digital system usable for viral exposure notification or contact tracing. While traditional contact tracing requires either that a person with a verified positive test informs people they have encountered or that medical professionals interview the infected person to infer what procedures are necessary to avoid further spread of the contagion, a DTTS makes it possible to immediately inform anyone using the system if they have been at risk of exposure. Such techniques can thus efficiently be used in a pandemic to ensure that exposed individuals are informed of a need to quarantine or get tested.

Parallel to these developments there are worries that authoritarian regimes, as well as democratically elected leaders with anti-democratic tendencies, will use the pandemic as a pretext to restrict human rights, increase surveillance, and ensure political control (IDEA 2020). According to a Freedom House Report 'COVID-19 has exacerbated the global decline in freedom. The outbreak exposed weaknesses across all the pillars of democracy, from elections and the rule of law to egregiously disproportionate restrictions on freedoms of assembly and movement' (Repucci and Slipowitz 2021: 10–11). In this context, DTTSs are particularly worrisome because they potentially offer a way to broadly monitor and control

Björn Lundgren, *Ethical Requirements for Digital Systems for Contact Tracing in Pandemics: A Solution to the Contextual Limits of Ethical Guidelines* In: *The Ethics of Surveillance in Times of Emergency.* Edited by: Kevin Macnish and Adam Henschke, Oxford University Press. © Oxford University Press 2023. DOI: 10.1093/oso/9780192864918.003.0011 a large collective of people. This raises the question of whether, and how, we can effectively combat the spread of a pandemic, while also safeguarding democratic values and fundamental human rights. The aim of this paper is to address this challenge, with respect to DTTSs.

Even when all parties are attempting to act conscientiously, DTTSs (just like vaccines and treatments) raise various ethical concerns, which must be properly addressed to minimize or avoid harm. The research community has been responsive to the basic challenge, by quickly providing ethical evaluation and guidelines for DTTSs (see, e.g., O'Neill et al. 2020; Klar and Lanzerath 2020; Lundgren 2020a; Morley et al. 2020; Raskar et al. 2020). The first aim of this chapter is to provide an extremely short set of ethical guidelines for the development and use of DTTSs. These guidelines build on work in Lundgren (2020a), which in turn criticized a pre-publication version of Morley et al. (2020). I picked their guidelines for several reasons. First, because amongst the early guidelines being proposed, Morley et al.'s are amongst the most usable, by which I mean that the ethical requirements are easily assessable by people who lack ethical expertise. Their brief and clear bivalent checklist can easily be evaluated without requiring ethical expertise. Second, amongst the early guidelines, they offered more analytical clarity than most.

Yet, despite their qualities there is plenty of room for improvements. First, while their guidelines are specifically intended for Covid-19, I aim to provide requirements that are useful in pandemics broadly. Second, while their guidelines are formulated as addressing requirements for *development* (even if they also address issues relating to *use*), I will provide requirements that can guide both *development* and *use* of DTTSs. Third, they focus on justifiability, while I will focus on permissibility, allowing me to further streamline and simplify the requirements. Indeed, the guidelines I propose depend on fewer requirements, which are formulated in a way that have much broader implications. Lastly, there is room for improvement in the sense that some prima facie sensible requirement should be jettisoned.

However, the arguably most interesting contribution in this chapter is not the specific guidelines as such, but the problems I raise for developing this kind of guidelines in general and my solution to those problems.[1] The guidelines that I develop in this chapter serve as an important example to the issues I raise in the penultimate section. In that section, I address a number of risks that create challenges for traditional guidelines. I see these risks as:

- the risk that implementing a DTTS solution changes informational distribution norms for the worse;

---

[1] I raised versions of these problems already in Lundgren (2020a), but I did not provide any solution.

- the risk that contextual factors change after implementing a DTTS solution, so that a specific DTTS solution becomes ethically inappropriate;
- the risk that the implementation of a DTTS solution in one country contributes to ethically detrimental policy applications in another country.

This chapter will be structured as follows. In the next section, I will introduce the ethical guidelines by Morley et al., which will serve as a way to critically assess my own proposal. In the following section, I present my own ethical requirements, which are extremely brief. The majority of the discussion is focused on explaining the implication of the limited requirements. A complete guideline needs to include such implication for useability. After this, I turn the discuss the above risks for ethical guidelines in general. Lastly, I will end the chapter by summarizing the main conclusions.

## Morley et al.'s Guidelines

In this section I describe Morley et al.'s guidelines. They consist of a set of sixteen yes/no questions, divided hierarchically into two parts. Each part is accompanied by an overarching question and each of the sixteen questions is complemented with a more detailed contextualization, which indicates that there is room for more gradual differences than the bivalent choices may indicate. Each answer indicates whether the system is more or less justifiable. Moreover, the ethical justifiability is also contextually dependent and may vary relative to different times and places.[2]

The first part of the guidelines consists of four questions, which they characterize as 'principles' in relation to the overarching question: 'is this the right app to develop?' (Morley et al. 2020: 30). These are:

1. 'Is it necessary?'
2. 'Is it proportionate?'
3. 'Is it sufficiently effective, timely, popular and accurate?'
4. 'Is it temporary?'

As previously noted, the yes/no answers to these questions are further specified in a way that explains how we should understand each question: making clear that whether the solution is necessary depends on whether it saves lives; that 'the gravity of the situation justifies the potential negative impact'; that there is

---

[2] For example, a smartphone app might work well in 'South Korea—where more than 95% of people owned a smartphone in 2018. But it might be less justifiable in Japan, where 66% of the population did.' (Morley et al. 2020: 31).

evidence to support its effectiveness etcetera; and that 'there is an explicit and reasonable date on which it will cease' (Morley et al. 2020: 30).

The second part of the guidelines, which they characterize as 'requirements', asks if the app is 'being developed in the right way?'. It consists of twelve questions in relation to the overarching question. As before, although all questions are binary, the answers add descriptions that contextualize and develop each of the twelve criteria. The questions ask (5) whether using the DTTS is *voluntary*, (6) whether *informed consent* is required, (7) whether 'privacy and users' anonymity is preserved', (8) whether there is a *self-erase function for user data*, (9) whether the *purpose of data collection is explicitly defined*, (10) whether the *purpose is limited*, (11) whether the system is *used only for prevention*, (12) whether the system avoids adding functionality of compliance, (13) whether the system is *open-source*, (14) whether the system is *equally available*, (15) *equally accessible*, and (16) whether there is *a decommission process for the system* (Morley et al. 2020: 30).

## My Proposed Guidelines

In this section, I will present and explain my alternative guidelines, using Morley et al. as the main comparative example (when the comparison does not raise any substantial issues, I just note in a footnote how my requirements cover theirs).

As noted in the Introduction, my guidelines formulate criteria for permissibility rather than justifiability.[3] On most standard ethical theory a DTTSs would be permissible only if all things considered, the good-making features of it outweigh its negative ethical impact.[4] While this may seem as a purely consequence-based consideration, we need not read 'good-making' or 'impact' as merely being constituted by consequences (e.g., an ethical impact can be a violation of someone's rights). Moreover, although my reasoning may be consequence-based, I am concerned with a plurality of values that often are associated with other ethical theories. Based on this we can formulate the following criterion:

BASIC PERMISSIBLITY CRITERION:    A DTTS is permissible only if, all things considered, our best estimate of its effectiveness (in reducing the spread of the

---

[3] While it may seem as if I am setting-aside an important issue at this stage—that is, how we choose between two permissible DTTSs—I will address that issue in the final section.

[4] This is in line with the view that ethics of machine decisions is a matter of trade-offs between the best output and the costs of achieving that output (Lundgren 2021).

virus through contact tracing) outweighs the risk—or possibility—of negative impacts.[5]

Henceforth, I will use the above requirement to see if there is a fundamental conflict between the aim of the DTTS (effective contact tracing) and the risks of negative impacts (e.g., human rights violations or bad outcomes). One may think this requires a further specification of how we ought to measure, or operationalize, *effectiveness*. However, on this issue I take no stance, because it depends partly on our ability to evaluate different suggested measurements. For example, estimating QALY will be extremely difficult for a disease such as Covid-19, since long-term effects are still unknown. That is, what I suggest is that it depends on the specific pandemic.[6]

   Moreover, I should note that I qualify this as a merely necessary criterion since we may, for example, have two DTTS systems that are equally effective but one has worse data protection, *ceteris paribus*. If so, then both systems cannot be permissible.

   With the permissibility criterion in place, the most important questions turn on the prima facie conflict between what information is needed to collect to make the DTTS efficient and the potential negative impacts of processing such data. The first criterion addresses questions of voluntariness and informed consent, after which I will turn to questions addressing the scope of data processing, and finally the question of equity of end-users' access.

CONSENT CRITERION:    A DTTS is permissible only if it satisfies a retractable informed consent, with the following exceptions: the consent requirement can be overridden in cases when a permissible non-DTTS alternative to ensure public health provides less or equal liberty and autonomy as the DTTS alternative and the DTTS is otherwise permissible.[7]

---

   [5] This criterion covers the three first principles from Morley et al. First, what is at stake in principle 3 is the effectiveness of the DTTS (e.g., questions concerning accuracy is just a means to an end, and evidence of effectiveness is just a question of our epistemic credence). Second, principle 2—whether the DTTS solution is proportionate—is captured by the above formulation, since it is a question of evaluating the benefits of the system against its potential negative impacts. Likewise, principle 1, the question of necessity—that is, whether we need the app in order to save lives—depends on the effectiveness of the DTTS. Thus, effectiveness is what is at stake.
   [6] Alternatives include, for example, the number of lives saved; the totality of qualitative life-years ('QALY') saved; reduction in transmission (i.e., reduction of the basic reproduction number, $R_0$); or the total number of people that can avoid risking exposure to the pandemic. I take here that the aim of a DTTS is to help improve public health. Alternatively, one could think that the efficiency measure should be defined in economic terms (for example). This is an interesting discussion that I have, because of page restrictions, set aside in this paper. Lastly, the choice of measurement may have some have informational costs (e.g., some kinds of measurement methods may be privacy invasive).
   [7] This overlaps with a few of Morley et al.'s requirements. First, (5) voluntariness and (6) that a consent can be withdrawn are directly covered in this criterion. Second, being informed also implies that (9) the purpose of data collection must be defined, and it also covers part of the goal of (13) open sources (i.e., allowing for inspection, p. 30).

An informed consent standardly requires *voluntariness, decisional capacity* and that the consenting party is *sufficiently and relevantly informed* (see, e.g., Eyal 2019). Thus, by 'consent requirement' I mean a requirement for decisionally capacitated voluntariness. Understood this way, consent can conflict directly with efficiency. Given that, in many cases, a larger the user base means a more efficient DTTS, an ability not to join can decrease efficiency. Similarly, we can worry about situations in which someone lacks decisional capacity, even if I presume that in most situations when someone lacks decisional capacity, someone else can consent for them.[8]

One might think that consent should be deemed less important because the impact of using a DTTS under strong data protection practices would be minimal. Yet, I have opted for pro tanto requiring consent because as I will argue in the next section, we have reason to opt for strong requirements that hold in any given context. Thus, consent is and should be a cornerstone criterion.

Nevertheless, we have to recognize that there are situations in which a consent requirement can and must be overridden (e.g., when the survival of mankind is at stake). The question we must address thus becomes a balancing act, which depends on the specific pandemic. In the case of Covid-19, a consent requirement should outweigh effectiveness—at least at a stage when vaccines effectively protect us against the most serious outcomes. Yet, we can imagine situations in which we are on the brink of catastrophic outcomes, in which a consent requirement can be overridden. Arguably, if infringement of liberty through quarantines can be permissible in the absence of a consent, then so can a DTTS under special circumstances Indeed, we standardly think that quarantine can be ethically permissible. For example, imagine the spread of a much more serious disease—such as a disease caused by a modified version of Ebola or the Marburg virus. In such situations, restriction on a consent requirement may become permissible or even obligatory. Hence, I suggest that the consent requirement is overridable.

One may think that the conditions under which public health overrides a consent requirement require further clarifications. However, this is not something I aim to solve here. Rather I fix the requirement based on such debates being solved elsewhere—for example, under which conditions a quarantine is permissible.[9]

Lastly, two limits to an *informed* consent should be noted. First, it is practically difficult to properly inform an individual of the potential consequences of sharing their data (see Nissenbaum 2011 for argument against consent; see also Ohm 2010; Lundgren 2020b for a discussion on the consequences of information and

---

[8] The most common example in which someone consents for someone else is parental consent (i.e., when parents consent for their child). While parental consent must be limited (see Elstub 2022), a DTTS system does not need to raise such worries in case we have sufficient data protection requirements in place.

[9] Of course, for full usability we need to explicate such conditions.

sharing). However, given that my proposed constraint for data usage is extremely limited this will be less of an issue. Second, a more pertinent problem is that consent agreements can create a 'red herring' or serve as a 'false flag' because they can make inappropriate information handling practices seem (more) appropriate. It is therefore important to keep in mind that requiring an informed consent says nothing about whether the consenting party *should* consent to the agreement, or even that it is an activity that is ethically permissible to consent to, which is why the next criterion is so important.

As mentioned above, some of the reasoning that underpins formulation of the consent criterion concerns what data is used and collected. Because aggregation of data and information is potentially sensitive, it matters how the data is processed. Thus, I suggest the following criterion:

DATA PROCESSING CRITERION: A DTTS is permissible only if data is handled in a way that ensures that it is only used, collected, created, or stored for the purpose of the DTTS (i.e., to determine risk of exposure by proximity to a verified or suspected carrier at a given time and date).

This criterion manages to balances efficiency against data protecting because it is forcefully restrictive without any substantial detriment to effectiveness (i.e., since the DTTS can collect precisely what is needed). However, the criterion has a few implication that may require clarification. First, given the defined purpose of a DTTS, data can only be used for prevention.[10] Second, it implies that *the data must be deleted when it no longer serves the given purpose.*[11]

This later implication requires a bit more discussion, since I have opted against end-users' ability to self-erase data.[12] Although self-erasure supports user autonomy, such a requirement is highly problematic since if end-users can delete specific data points this would directly reduce efficiency (especially if many users delete data points that overlap in space and time). Thus, erase functions require a balancing act. On my reasoning a requirement that user data be automatically deleted when it no longer satisfies the purpose would suffice. Consider the fact that contact tracing in most pandemics requires only a limited set of data for a limited time period.

---

[10]  Cf. Morley et al. (2020), requirement 11.

[11]  This makes two of Morley et al.'s (2020) criteria redundant. According to principle 4 'there is an explicit and reasonable date on which it will cease' (p. 30). While such a requirement cannot be practically satisfied given that it is practically impossible to foresee when a pandemic will be over, it is also redundant given that data will be deleted when no longer useful. The same type of redundancy reasoning also applies to requirement 16, since there is no need for a 'decommissioning process' (p. 30) if there is no data to be deleted.

[12]  Cf. Morley et al. (2020), requirement 8.

Nevertheless, one may worry that our spatio-temporal locations may reveal a lot more about us.[13] However, there is no need to worry about *locations* since they need not be collected or stored. All the spatio-temporal information that is needed is that individual A and B are in the same location at a given date and time. Thus, a third implication of the requirement is that *locational data can only be used, collected, created, or stored for the purpose of determining that two individuals are in the same location (where that location cannot be used, collected, created, or stored)*. All that needs to be added to create a functioning DTTS is test results (or to allow end-users to add symptoms, in the absence of reliable testing). Moreover, granted that the data can only be accessed for the given purpose, users' privacy and anonymity worries are limited for most pandemics.

However, there are some complicated cases that merit further discussion. Suppose a DTTS required collection of more sensitive data. For example, what if one wanted to use a DTTS for a sexually transmitted infection. As I have defined the data processing criterion, collecting information about sexual contacts is not permissible. Whether that on balance is motivated, vis-à-vis the basic permissibility criterion, is partly an empirical question, but as will be seen in the next section, the strict data processing criterion is motivated on the ground of the risks raised in the Introduction.

Another example has to do with a broader purpose, such as studying data patterns. For example, studying *where* spreading occurs may be very helpful to create advice and best practices for minimizing the spread of the virus. As is clear from a previous clarification, this is not permissible (since locations cannot be processed in this way). There are various reasons why it should not be permitted, but the simplest explanation is that this is not a purpose for a DTTS. Why? Because it is not about tracing and tracking, it is an open-ended (scientific) investigation, which requires a different set of ethical considerations.[14] In particular, scientific investigations raise special research ethical concerns. For a DTTS the data collection must be limited, since the data and informational risks are otherwise too substantial. The risk is not only about individuals but also about collective harms, such as our democracy (see, e.g. Ohm 2010; Lundgren 2020b; van den Hoven 1997; Véliz 2020). Another example of non-individual harm is a local business that becomes associated with disease-spreading (Raskar et al. 2020: 8).

In this context it is worthwhile discussing the use of differential privacy (promoted by Morley et al. promotes, see requirement 7). This is an odd idea, since the goal of differential privacy is to protect privacy by ensuring that the data is anonymous and making it impossible to re-identify the user based on the

---

[13] For example, consider how certain locations may be sensitive (e.g., a woman's shelter, health clinic, therapist). Moreover, in Lundgren (2020b) I argue that these types of patterns—whether linked to us or not—would reduce our ability to be anonymous (i.e., our ability to maintain anonymity in any given situation), because it makes deanonymization (or reidentification) easier.

[14] Cf. Morley et al. (2020), requirement 11.

dataset (see, e.g., Dwork and Roth 2014). That is, if we use differential privacy, then the DTTS will become useless (because it will be impossible to identify a given user in the dataset and thus inform them of the risk of exposure). However, for other kind of systems, for example, those set-up for the purpose of studying disease patterns, differential privacy may prove useful. Even if it would not resolve all data-related worries (cf. Lundgren 2020b).

This takes us to the fourth implication of the data processing criterion: That *data cannot be stored in a way that depend on user's own security standard.*[15] This contradicts Morley et al., who opt for storing data locally. Contrarily, given that an end-user of a DTTS should not be held *morally* responsible for securing her data, a requirement that data be stored locally is arguably problematic because it shifts causal responsibility in a way that mismatches with the moral responsibility (Lundgren 2020a). That is, the security of data on an end-user's device depends partly on the end-user, which is also a worry in itself. Since the data processing criterion requires that access is *ensured*, this implies that the data must be secured by the DTTS provider (see Lundgren and Möller 2019 for an analysis and definition of information security).

Issues of security also relate to questions of *open source* (Morley et al., requirement 13). Arguably, open-source should be viewed as a means to an end to *enable code evaluation*—to protect against mistakes and malicious code, and to achieve the best possible code (e.g., through collaboration). That is, we should not necessarily require open source, but that there is a *way to verify and evaluate the code* (Lundgren 2020a). Whether we ought to require verification depends on whether it is technically possible and if it can efficiently be achieved. If it can, then we could modify the data processing criterion to require verifiability (if possible).

Fifth, and finally, the limits of data usage also mean that a DTTS cannot be used for compliance or for other purposes, since it is restricted to a limited usage.[16]

Now that I've dealt with the conditions of accepting the use of the system and the rules for data practices, the final requirement concerns access to, and availability of, the system:

END-USER ACCESS:   A DTTS is permissible only if it is available to and compatible with access for all end-users.

This requirement is both about equity and effectiveness. Here it is important to distinguish between whether an application is *available* to all end-users and whether they have the technical means to *access* it (cf. Morley et al.). The effectiveness of a DTTS increases if it is available and accessible to all. Although

---

[15] If data security depends on the end users' own secure standard, then the requirements about ensuring limits to data processing cannot be satisfied.
[16] Cf. Morley et al. (2020), requirement 10 and 12.

access to some may prove costly, it is difficult to imagine a realistic scenario in which it would be beneficial to restrict access to a small subgroup (i.e., conflict with *availability*). Even if we could think of a situation in which a particular group is *prioritized* for various reasons (e.g., the state may be motived to prioritize medical personnel when it comes to limited access to vaccination and testing capabilities, to ensure that safety of medical treatments for patients and that the medical system does not crash). However, even in such special cases this priority would not conflict with the underlying value of equality (because prioritizing medical personal would be done for the benefit of all people).[17] Note also that it is 'compatible with access' because requiring access for all is too strong. Simply put, in practice we cannot *ensure* access for all, but neither should a DTTS be designed to deny access.

To sum up, I have defended a streamlined set of ethical requirements that explains when a DTTS is permissible. These concern voluntariness and consent, data practices, and equitable end-user access. I have done so by making use of the basic permissibility criterion, which stated that a DTTS is permissible only if the efficiency outweighs the potential negative impacts. Furthermore, I have presented and defended various more specific implications of the limited requirements (using Morley et al. as a critical counterpoint). Lastly, each criterion is necessary and they are jointly sufficient, with one caveat: I have said nothing about how we choose between two, or more, prima facie permissible systems. That is, what the criteria jointly identifies is a set containing the permissible system(s). In case the set includes more than one system, the choice is sometimes obvious (e.g., one has stronger data protection than another, *ceteris paribus*, or one is more effective than the other, *ceteris paribus*) but some of these choices may include trade-offs. I will address this issue at least partially in the following section.

## How to Protect against Contextual Change

In this section, I will start by discussing and describing the risks that I listed in the introduction. That is: (1) the risk that broad usage of a DTTS changes social or societal norms for the worse; (2) the risk that the context which makes a DTTS ethically permissible changes so that it is no longer ethically permissible; and (3) the risk that the implementation of a good DTTS solution in one country contributes to ethically detrimental policy applications in another country.

---

[17] We might also have reasons to focus on *risk groups*, for which the above argument *prima facie* may seem less applicable. However, protecting risk groups can be beneficial for everyone, because it preserves medical resources (a serious problem during the current pandemic has arguably been access to medical resources). How one should prioritize resources between different groups is a discussion that I must set aside due to the word limit (see, e.g., Parfit 1997).

The first substantial question I want to address is whether these risks can be solved within standard ethical guidelines. In addressing this issue, I will also see if we can qualify what kind of risks these are. Next, I will sketch an idea on how to resolve or mitigate these problems. This solution also raises the question of how to choose between alternative systems (which the requirements in the previous sections ignore).

The first risk (i.e., that DTTS could changes social norms for the worse) could be formulated as a slippery slope. If implementing a DTTS leads to a chain of events that eventually results in a worse situation.[18] That is, temporary measures can affect and change societal and social norms for the worse (e.g., consider how social media has changed individuals' norms of information distribution). However, the risk I envision here can also simply be a risk actualized because temporary measures become permanent (see, e.g., Rentoul 2018 for a few illustrative examples). The second risk (i.e., that the context changes, so that the DTTS should no longer be considered permissible), is about substantial contextual change (e.g., in the political landscape) while a DTTS measure is in place so that what is appropriate changes (e.g., if a less democratic party or leader ascends). Because these ethical guidelines are contextually sensitive it can be difficult to handle contextual changes that are caused by the DTTS or happen while the system is used. Moreover, the third risk (i.e., the risk that implementation of a DTTS has negative effects elsewhere) goes beyond the context in which the DTTS is normally implemented. That is, the risk that choices made by one country can affect the choices made in *other countries*. Consider, for example, how Trump's rhetoric about the media has spread to, and been used by, oppressive regimes (see, e.g., Schwartz 2018). That is, the implementation of policies in a democratic country—policies that are appropriate in a democratic nation, but not in an oppressive regime—may supply an undemocratic regime with a reason to adopt the same policy. Moreover, even *good choices* in liberal democracies can influence *bad choices* in less liberal regimes. That is, usage of DTTSs in democratic countries can be used as a pretext for using abusive systems that are, or are presented as, DTTSs but also serve other means (e.g., mass surveillance). More broadly, we need to consider how policy choices in one nation affect policy choices in other nations.[19]

The best way to qualify these risks and explain why they fall somewhat outside of the scope of the ordinary guidelines is that they are risks that affect or are affected by the context. Granted that any technology must be analysed

---

[18] For discussions on the validity of slippery slope arguments (see, e.g., van der Burg 1991; Hansen 2020).

[19] If one considers the decision to use a DTTS a national decision, then one could potentially question to what extent a nation is responsible for the actions of other nations. However, even if we think that responsibility is somehow limited by national boundaries, it is arguably worse for a democratic nation if other nations become less democratic.

in context, including DTTSs—that is, the justifiability and permissibility of a DTTS is contextually sensitive—it follows that these risks are difficult to address in standard guidelines. The type of checklist that Morley et al. use cannot easily address risks that are due to more substantial contextual change (e.g., such that the ethical analysis does not longer apply).

Granted this challenge, how do we to protect against or mitigate these risks? I will suggest an ideal solution, which is quite simple: there should be *one* DTTS and it should be developed under the control of a trustworthy international organization with relevant medical (and ethical) expertise. (NB, what organization satisfies these demands is partly an empirical question, which I am not in a position to judge. However, to my mind, the kind of organization that we should look for can be exemplified by the *World Health Organization*.)

There are some prima facie obvious problems with this solution (e.g., how could countries with different desires plausibly agree on an international tool?). I will address such and other worries as I explain and explicate the solution. That is, despite the fact that the solution may prima facie seem as a one size fits all solution, I will show how there is room for pluralism.

The solution addresses the risks in various ways. First, if we settle for *one global DTTS*, then this would resolve part of the third risk (i.e., that authoritarian regimes motivate or whitewashes the use of an unscrupulous or entirely unethical system, because of other kinds of DTTSs are being used elsewhere).[20]

Second, the remaining variant of the third risk as well as the second risk can be resolved if we can develop a system that is ethically appropriate in a variety of contexts. This can arguably be achieved if we adopt a standard of protection of human rights and values that is suitable for the *worst possible context*.[21] As long as the DTTS satisfies the permissibility criterion, this would be a sensible solution given that it does not imply any increased risk of negative impacts in other contexts.

Third, by adapting strong protections of fundamental values, we also protect against the first risk. If the DTTS adheres to appropriate norms (i.e., ethical norms, as identified in the guidelines), then there is less risk that it can change norms for the worse.

Lastly, adhering to strong protection of fundamental values also gives us an idea on how we should choose between alternative DTTS solutions. For example, we

---

[20] Of course, even if international cooperation results in the broad use of *one* DTTS, there is a risk that authoritarian regimes use the existence of that one system as a reason for developing their own (e.g., by criticizing international democratic cooperation). Yet, it would be more difficult to motivate their own system on the basis of everyone else using *one* and the *same* system. Because it takes away the basic argument that everyone else has their *own* system.

[21] One may worry that this would hamper efficiency. However, it is important to keep in mind that the basic permissibility criterion still is in place. Moreover, what I hope to have shown in the previous section is that a lot of *prime facie* conflicts between efficiency and negative impacts can be resolved, without severe degradation of the systems efficiency.

should enact strong data protection principles, while still ensuring that the DTTS solution is permissible. My hope is that the previous section provides at least an idea of how this can be satisfied. Despite a potential need for a more applied analysis (e.g., to determine further implications and settle some of the unresolved issues from the previous section), it is clear that once we have determined what is needed in response to the worst possible context, we should aim for a DTTS that is as efficient as possible given those requirements.[22]

Beyond solving the three risks, using one DTTS also creates various benefits and can be motivated based on the permissibility criteria. Arguably, a plurality of systems would be less *justifiable* because it would decrease efficiency (unless there is a joint data sharing) and because it increases the risk of abuse. Hence, using one system seems to be motivated both on the grounds that it would increase efficiency and because it can minimize the negative impacts.[23]

This solution also raises a number of issues and potential counterarguments. Even if all details cannot be discussed here, some of these warrant brief comment. Broadly, there are at least six practical challenges: (1) Does the solution complicate the ethical analysis? (2) How can one DTTS solution work when the user base is so diverse? (3) How can we have *one* DTTS solution for different pandemics? (4) What are the fallbacks if this type of international collaboration around one system is not achievable? (5) How do we deal with other DTTSs? (6) By focusing on *one* system, are we not missing the positive benefits of competition?

First, it may seem as if the solution complicates the ethical evaluation because we have to look to what is required in the worst possible context (which explains why the requirement I formulated in the previous section aimed to be fairly strict). Given the aim that ethical guidelines should be usable by non-experts we have to look for ways to reduce that complexity. Surely, it is simpler to look to one's own context, but the effort is helped and simplified by international collaboration and by letting a trustworthy international organization deal with the data handling. In addition, all things considered, the total analytic complexity is arguably reduced by having only one system. Moreover, the requirements presented in the previous section do not pose any significant problem, even if we could imagine a more liberal set of requirements being suitable in some contexts.

Second, an international user base is clearly much more diverse than a national one—for example, relative to access to smartphone devices, stable Internet connections, and digital literacy. One solution to this would be to make different versions of the application available. While this may seem like a contradiction, it is not. The point here is that there should by one DTT *system*, which is in no way

---

[22] I hope this idea explains why I opted for relatively strict requirements in the previous section. Also, cf. fn. 21 for worries about efficiency.

[23] There may be special reasons to require special approaches in special limited cases (such as for personal at hospitals), but that is a different question.

incompatible with making it available on different platforms or making versions that are more suitable in contexts of limited internet connections (e.g., this may require temporally extended local storage of data, which otherwise should be avoided). Again, there is some pluralism in this solution, despite the fact that it may seem as if I first intended that one size fits all.

Third, given that we might need different systems for different pandemics, what we want is an *overall architecture for DTTSs*. This architecture should be used to create a—that is, one—specific DTTS for a specific pandemic. That is, we should develop a *meta-system* that can be modified in different ways, depending on how we evaluate the balancing act relative to different criteria and different viruses. That meta-system is the architecture; a specific system is one way in which that architecture can be set; and a DTTS application is the end-user device.

Fourth, achieving international collaboration around one system can be difficult. Thus, we have to discuss what we should do in cases when it is not feasible to achieve such international collaboration and coordination. If international agreement on a joint DTTS project is not possible, the responsible international organization should still aim to develop a DTTS in accordance with the suggested ethical criteria and then aim to promote that system (i.e., the aim should be to achieve one system that is as widely accepted as possible). Alternatively, if the international organization is not in a position to develop a DTTS, the aim should be to agree upon joint technical and ethical standards (preferably in accordance with criteria suggested here).

Fifth, related to joint technical and ethical standards, if there are more systems in use, then how should the system we have developed deal with the presence of other systems? On the one hand, to increase efficiency it may seem as if one should opt for data input from other systems. Yet, on the other hand, if one cannot verify a sufficient quality for the data from other systems, then using that data may be detrimental (e.g., because it may reduce trust in our system or result in unnecessary and detrimental choices). Moreover, one should not share data with other systems unless we can verify that these systems maintain an appropriate ethical standard. Sharing data puts the data at risk, which defeats the whole balancing act and may make our system impermissible if the parties with whom we share the data handle it inappropriately. Thus, in most situations one only want an input from other systems (with no, or extremely limited, output).[24] This, again, shows that one joint solution is to be preferred—especially if we are talking of a scenario when we want to enable travel over national borders (given global trading and

---

[24] Here it is interesting to consider that the EU has set up a protocol for data-sharing between national apps within the EU. This is a variant of what I propose. It does not offer one architecture, but a joint data-sharing framework.

goods transportation, nation crossing will arguably be necessary in many scenarios).

Sixth, one prima facie benefit of using many systems is the ability to find optimal solutions through market competition, which may also enable us to learn from market-experimentation. Yet, there is nothing in my proposal that forbids market competition. What I suggest, however, is that the market should be direct towards one customer: the international organization. Hence, despite starting off with a prima facie monistic solution (i.e., one size fits all), I hope to have shown how that idea is compatible with pluralism to resolve the problems related to having one size fit all in a diverse global context.

## Conclusion

In the first part of this chapter, I proposed a set of ethical requirements for permissibility of DTTS solutions. Since I focused on permissibility, rather than justifiability, it pushed the question of how we choose between alternative permissible DTTSs—should we prioritize protection against negative impacts or focus on efficiency? This question depends on the context of where the DTTS solution is applied. In the final part of the chapter, I answered this question by addressing an overarching problem for ethical guidelines: context change. I argued that we should focus on the worst possible context (i.e., the context that requires the most protections against negative impacts). Moreover, I argued that although it may seem as if that would reduce efficiency, because I suggest that we should have *one* DTT system (for each pandemic and *one* DTTS architecture that can be adapted for a specific pandemic), it arguably follows that such a solution would increase efficiency (and have various border-crossing benefits). I also argued that this solution would resolve the risks of contextual change, because there would be one system for all countries, one system that is conservative enough not to challenge any good norms, and one system that would be appropriate in all contexts. Lastly, I argued that despite having one system for all contexts, we can have different applications that are adapted to various contextual differences (while the system's protection against negative impacts remains the same).[25]

[25] I want to thank Karim Jebari, Kalle Grill, and attendances at the higher seminar in philosophy at the Royal Institute of Technology (Stockholm, Sweden) for helpful comments on earlier drafts, and Joel Anderson and Sven Nyholm for a helpful discussion during the final revisions. I also want to thank the editors of, and the reviewers for, this anthology. Lastly, I want to acknowledge that this work was supported by the Wallenberg AI, Autonomous Systems and Software Program—Humanities and Society (WASP-HS) funded by the Marianne and Marcus Wallenberg Foundation and the Marcus and Amalia Wallenberg Foundation (grant number: MMW 2018.0116). The work was also supported by and part of the research programme Ethics of Socially Disruptive Technologies, which is funded through the Gravitation programme of the Dutch Ministry of Education, Culture, and Science and the Netherlands Organization for Scientific Research (NWO grant number 024.004.031).

# References

Dwork, C. and A. Roth. 2014. 'The Algorithmic Foundations of Differential Privacy'. *Theoretical Computer Science* 9 (3–4): 211–407. https://doi.org/10.1561/0400000042.

Elstub, E. 2022. *Surveillance Capitalism: The Harm to Childhood, the Insufficiency of Parental Consent and the Consequent Impermissibility.* MA thesis, Utrecht University.

Eyal, N. 2019. 'Informed Consent'. In *The Stanford Encyclopedia of Philosophy.* Spring 2019 Edition. https://plato.stanford.edu/archives/spr2019/entries/informed-consent/.

Hansen, H. 2020. 'Fallacies'. In *The Stanford Encyclopedia of Philosophy.* Summer 2020 Edition. https://plato.stanford.edu/archives/sum2020/entries/fallacies/.

IDEA (The International Institute for Democracy and Electoral Assistance). 2020. A Call to Defend Democracy. June 25. Retrieved from: https://www.idea.int/news-media/multimedia-reports/call-defend-democracy.

Klar, R. and D. Lanzerath. 2020. 'The Ethics of COVID-19 Tracking Apps—Challenges and Voluntariness'. *Research Ethics* 16 (3–4): 1–9. https://doi.org/10.1177/1747016120943622.

Lundgren, B. 2020a. 'Improving on and Assessing Ethical Guidelines for Digital Tracking and Tracing Systems for Pandemics'. *Ethics and Information Technology.* https://doi.org/10.1007/s10676-020-09561-z.

Lundgren, B. 2020b. 'Beyond the Concept of Anonymity: What Is Really at Stake?' In *Big Data and Democracy*, edited by K. Macnish and J. Galliot, 201–16. Edinburgh: Edinburgh University Press. https://edinburghuniversitypress.com/pub/media/resources/9781474463522_Chapter_13.pdf.

Lundgren, B. 2021. 'Ethical Machine Decisions and the Input-Selection Problem'. *Synthese* 199: 11423–43. https://doi.org/10.1007/s11229-021-03296-0.

Lundgren, B. and N. Möller. 2019. 'Defining Information Security'. *Science Engineering Ethics* 25: 419–41. https://doi.org/10.1007/s11948-017-9992-1.

Morley, J., J. Cowls, M. Taddeo, and L. Floridi. 2020. 'Ethical Guidelines for COVID-19 Tracing Apps'. *Nature* 582: 29–31. https://doi.org/10.1038/d41586-020-01578-0.

Nissenbaum, H. 2011. 'A Contextual Approach to Privacy Online'. *Dædalus, the Journal of the American Academy of Arts & Sciences* 140 (4): 32–48. https://doi.org/10.1162/DAED_a_00113.

Ohm, P. 2010. 'Broken Promises of Privacy: Responding to the Surprising Failure of Anonymization'. *UCLA Law Rev* 57: 1701–77. https://ssrn.com/abstract=1450006.

O'Neill, P. H., T. Ryan-Mosley, and B. Johnson. 2020. 'A Flood of Coronavirus Apps Are Tracking Us. Now It's Time to Keep Track of Them'. *MIT Technology Review*, 7 May. https://www.technologyreview.com/2020/05/07/1000961/launching-mittr-covid-tracing-tracker/.

Parfit, D. 1997. 'Equality and Priority'. *Ratio* 10 (3): 202–21. https://doi.org/10.1111/1467-9329.00041.

Raskar, R. et al. 2020. 'Apps Gone Rogue: Maintaining Personal Privacy in an Epidemic'. MIT White Paper. https://arxiv.org/abs/2003.08567.

Rentoul, J. 2018. 'The Top 10: Temporary Things That Turned Out to Be Permanent'. *Independent*, 30 June. https://www.independent.co.uk/voices/top-10-temporary-things-that-turned-out-to-be-permanent-a8421381.html.

Repucci, S. and Slipowitz. 2021. 'Freedom in the World 2021. Democracy under Siege'. Freedom House. https://freedomhouse.org/sites/default/files/2021-02/FIW2021_World_02252021_FINAL-web-upload.pdf

Schwartz, J. 2018. 'Trump's "Fake News" Rhetoric Crops up around the Globe'. *Politico*, 31 July. https://www.politico.eu/blogs/on-media/2018/07/donald-trump-fake-news-rhetoric-crops-up-around-the-globe-media-social-media-foreign-affairs/.

Van der Burg, W. 1991. 'The Slippery Slope Argument'. *Ethics* 102 (1): 42–65. https://doi.org/10.1086/293369.

van den Hoven, M. J. 1997. 'Privacy and The Varieties of Moral Wrong-Doing in an Information Age'. *SIGCAS Comput. Soc.* 27 (3): 33–7. https://doi.org/10.1145/270858.270868

Véliz, C. 2020. *Privacy is Power: Why and How You Should Take Back Control of Your Data*. London: Bantam Press.

# 11

# An Unexceptional Theory of Morally Proportional Surveillance in Exceptional Circumstances

*Frej Klem Thomsen*

How much surveillance is morally permissible in the pursuit of a socially desirable goal? Almost everyone agrees that there are limits to the amount of surveillance to which we can permissibly subject persons. Most also believe that the amount of permissible surveillance increases to the extent that the surveillance promotes a socially desirable goal. It makes a difference, for example, if surveillance can help prevent crime or improve health, and whether it can help to do so a little or a lot. Beyond these minimal points of consensus, however, opinions rapidly diverge. Specifically, there is widespread disagreement on the question of how to weigh the balance between the badness of surveillance and the achievement of socially desirable goals. How *exactly* does promoting a socially desirable goal by a certain amount affect the amount of morally permissible surveillance? Call this **the proportionality question of morally permissible surveillance.**[1]

The proportionality question drew renewed attention during the 2020 Coronavirus pandemic, because governments in many countries responded by implementing, redirecting, or expanding state surveillance, most controversially in the shape of collection and use of cell-phone location data to support a strategy of contact tracing, testing and containment.[2] (Ferretti et al. 2020; Singer and Sang-Hun 2020; The European Commission 2020) These initiatives drew vocal criticism, much of it focused on claims that increased surveillance was or would be disproportional (7amleh—Arab Center for Social Media Advancement et al. 2020; Morley, Cowls, Taddeo, and Floridi 2020; Stanley and Granick 2020).

---

[1] A closely related debate concerns the *legality* of increased surveillance. There may, however, be forms of surveillance, that are morally impermissible but legal and vice versa. Consideration of which types of surveillance are and ought to be legal is a separate matter. In the present I shall focus only on the question of moral permissibility.

[2] Such surveillance is, again, nothing new. Logging of cell-phone location data is an established practice in many countries. In the EU, for example, it has continued despite sustained criticism by civil rights organizations and being ruled illegal by the ECJ in 2016 (Brown and Korff 2009; European Court of Justice 2016).

Frej Klem Thomsen, *An Unexceptional Theory of Morally Proportional Surveillance in Exceptional Circumstances* In: *The Ethics of Surveillance in Times of Emergency.* Edited by: Kevin Macnish and Adam Henschke, Oxford University Press.
© Oxford University Press 2023. DOI: 10.1093/oso/9780192864918.003.0012

In response to such concerns, surveillance proponents have pointed to the fact that the Coronavirus pandemic constituted an exceptional global health emergency, and explicitly or implicitly claimed that circumstances justify surveillance measures that would ordinarily be impermissible. The French Digital Minister Cédric O defended use of the StopCovid contact tracing app, explaining that: 'StopCovid is not a "peacetime" app. Such a project would not exist without the situation created by Covid-19', because a restart of the epidemic could have 'catastrophic health, economic, social and democratic consequences. [...] It is under these conditions—and under these conditions only—that deployment of this application is envisaged by the government' (O 2020, my translation). Similarly, the Israeli Minister of Justice Amir Ohana responded to criticism of emergency surveillance conducted by Israeli intelligence service Shin Bet by stating that: 'The concerns of those disturbed by cyber monitoring are outweighed by the threat we are facing' (Heller 2020). Even more directly, in the UK, a report by the Tony Blair Institute concluded that:

> The price of [escape from the choice between protecting lives and protecting the economy] is an unprecedented increase in digital surveillance. In normal times the degree of monitoring and state intervention we are talking about here would be out of the question in liberal democracies. But these are not normal times, and the alternatives are even more unpalatable.
>
> (Bamford, Dace, Macon-Cooney, and Yiu 2020)

These responses highlight an issue behind the proportionality question, which is often overlooked. In fact, it seems to me that disagreements regarding the proportionality of surveillance in exceptional circumstances often turn on underlying disagreements about this issue. The issue is this: in what way does a state of emergency affect the proportionality of morally permissible surveillance? The question may seem trivial, but two very different answers are possible, and the choice between them has radical implications for how we must answer the proportionality question.

On one view, a state of emergency has the effect of suspending or altering at least some of the constraints on morally permissible (state) action that apply under ordinary circumstances. Let us call the application of this view to the proportionality question **the qualitative difference view** of proportional surveillance in a state of emergency (this view is expanded and explained below). On the qualitative difference view, there is a certain threshold, where the stakes become so great that the proportionality condition itself changes, either by becoming altogether void, or (more plausibly) by allowing greater amounts of surveillance relative to the social good achieved.

On another view, the only difference between states of emergency and ordinary circumstances is that the stakes are greater in a state of emergency. Let us call this the quantitative difference view of proportional surveillance in a state of emergency. On the quantitative difference view, morally proportional surveillance is a continuous, strictly increasing function of the social goods achieved by surveillance.

The difference between the two views is hopefully clear. If the qualitative difference view is true, then there are situations, perhaps such as 'the War on Terror' or the Coronavirus pandemic, during which the ordinary proportionality condition does not apply. If a proportionality condition applies at all, it requires a much less demanding ratio between social goods achieved and the badness of the surveillance performed. On the quantitative difference view, on the other hand, the proportionality condition applies in exactly the same way in a state of emergency as in ordinary circumstances. The only difference is that the stakes are higher, i.e., that the goods achieved through surveillance are greater, but the way we balance the badness of surveillance against these goods is unchanged.

The overall objective of this article is to argue against the qualitative and for the quantitative difference view. I proceed by first setting out in somewhat greater detail how we must understand the qualitative difference view (section two). I then present a series of problematic implications of adopting the qualitative difference view and argue that jointly these give us sufficient reason to reject it (section three). This entails that our account of morally permissible surveillance should be unexceptional, i.e., the quantitative difference view: there is no morally significant difference between proportionality in ordinary circumstances and proportionality in emergencies, simply a spectrum of smaller to greater potential goods and bads of surveillance. In order to flesh out the implications of the quantitative view, I briefly sketch an unexceptional theory of proportional surveillance in exceptional circumstances (section four). The last section (five) summarizes and concludes.

## The Qualitative Difference View of Proportional Surveillance in Exceptional Circumstances

The fundamental issue at stake in this chapter is how to specify our theory of morally proportional surveillance, particularly as it pertains to the difference between ordinary circumstances and a state of emergency. In this section, I will first set out in more detail what a condition of proportionality for morally permissible surveillance might look like on the qualitative difference view. I next motivate the qualitative difference view by illustrating how it resembles recognized positions in the literature. This sets the stage for the next section, in which I present a series of objections to the qualitative difference view.

The qualitative difference view as I have sketched it above is the idea that, in certain exceptional circumstances, the proportionality condition for morally permissible surveillance changes to allow forms or amounts of surveillance that would otherwise be disproportional. In a state of emergency, the view holds, there are moral exceptions. More precisely, I will say that **the qualitative difference view of proportionality for morally permissible surveillance** holds that:

(1) There is some threshold $T$, for the goods achieved by surveillance (e.g., averting or alleviating the effects of a global pandemic), where the proportionality condition changes.

(2) an act $\phi$ of surveillance is proportional in the sense relevant to moral permissibility *below* T *iff* the ratio of the goods that $\phi$'ing brings about over the bads that $\phi$'ing brings about is equal to or greater than some constant $k_1$, where $k_1$ is greater than 1:1 (e.g., 2:1, 3:2, 4:3, etc.).

(3) an act $\phi$ of surveillance is proportional in the sense relevant to moral permissibility *at or above* T *iff* the ratio of the goods that $\phi$'ing brings about over the bads that $\phi$'ing brings about is equal to or greater than some constant $k_2$, where $k_2$ is (much) smaller than $k_1$ but equal to or greater than 1:1.

Let me clarify four features of the definition. First, the ratios are required to be equal to or greater than one in order to ensure that proportionality requires as a bare minimum that the act does more good than bad. $k_1$ specifically must be not merely equal to but greater than one to allow for the possibility that $k_2$ is equal to one. Beyond these requirements, however, there can be different views on what the proper ratios for proportionality are.

Second, I assume that actions that bring about *no* bads need not satisfy a proportionality condition. While independently plausible—surely proportionality is only a requirement of actions that bring about at least *some* bads—this also ensures that we will never encounter a fraction with zero in the divisor (cf. Thomsen, 2020, pp. 21–22, discussing a requirement of surplus goods).

Third, I speak generically of the 'goods' and 'bads' that surveillance brings about, as placeholders for the values that go into weighing proportionality. In the context of e.g., public health surveillance these might be (very broadly) increased health on the one side (goods) and decreased privacy on the other (bads). I assume that goods and bads are in principle quantifiable and comparable—else how would we asses proportionality in the first place?—but I shall touch upon the details only briefly in section four below.

Fourth, the view is neutral with respect to the role of intentions for proportionality. It is commonly held in e.g., just war theory, that there is a significant difference between intentionally and foreseeably bringing about goods and bads. The qualitative view as stated above is compatible with this role for intentions, but also with denying that intentions (or mental states more broadly) affect proportionality. I invite the reader to assume that the discussion is focused on her preferred version among these two views.

What are we to think of the qualitative difference view? The notion of moral exceptions in exceptional circumstances is neither novel nor specific to the context of surveillance of public health. Perhaps most obviously, the qualitative difference view is related to or—given a suitably expansive definition—a form of threshold deontology. Threshold deontology posits that there are moral thresholds, where the consequences of an action outweigh or cancel the moral constraint, making the otherwise prohibited action morally permissible (Alexander 2000; Arneson 2018; Kagan 1988: 81–2). Thresholds for moral constraints can be defined either absolutely, for example for each separate act type, or relative to some variable value. If threshold deontology is understood as imposing a single constraint with a relative threshold on all actions, i.e., to require a certain ratio between the badness of the action (e.g., harm done or rights violated) and the resulting benefits (e.g., harm to others prevented), then it essentially becomes a principle of proportionality (Cf. Thomsen 2020).

This is not an implausible interpretation of threshold deontology, but it is not the only plausible interpretation of it either. More importantly, it is not the qualitative view. For it to be the qualitative view, the theory would have to hold that there is also a secondary threshold, where the resulting benefits are so great that the required ratio between the badness of the action and the resulting benefits changes (qua condition 3 in our definition above). Perhaps this view can be labelled a form of threshold deontology, but if so certainly a non-standard form.

Can the qualitative view draw on motivations for threshold deontology? Not directly. Standard threshold deontology is to a large degree motivated as a theoretical response to absolutist deontology. Absolutist deontology holds that there are moral constraints on at least some actions, which makes them morally impermissible regardless of circumstances. In Kant's notorious example, lying is morally wrong even when a murderer asks about the location of a prospective victim (Kant 1797, 1993). This, of course, is wildly implausible, and the ability to avoid such counter-intuitive implications is arguably the central attraction of threshold deontology. The qualitative view cannot directly draw on this motivation, because to avoid the pitfalls of absolutist deontology one needs only the standard threshold. However, the qualitative view can perhaps draw some indirect support from the general thrust of the argument for threshold deontology. Just as it is counterintuitive, some might say, that the scope of the consequences make no difference to moral constraints, even when the consequences are disastrous, so it is counterintuitive that the size of the stakes does not matter for proportionality, even when the stakes are enormous.

This thrust of argument is also at play in a second, perhaps more promising source of support. Within surveillance ethics, the increasingly sophisticated discussion of moral proportionality in recent years has utilized concepts and arguments developed in the just war theory literature (Henschke 2018; Macnish 2015, 2018; Rønn and Lippert-Rasmussen 2020; Thomsen 2020). That literature also hosts an extensive debate on the idea of moral exceptions in times of emergency. The most prominent defender of the idea of moral exceptions is Michael Walzer, who has argued that there can exist 'supreme emergencies', under which we may set aside at least some of the *jus in bello* constraints that ordinarily impose limits on morally permissible action in war[3] (Walzer 1977). Specifically, Walzer claims that it may in such situations be morally permissible to intentionally harm innocents to avert the threat.

The idea of supreme emergency as developed in just war theory does not, of course, transfer directly to the present context. The three most important differences are that the just war theory of moral exceptions under supreme emergencies (a) applies to antagonistic threats, i.e., to situations where great harm is threatened by an agent intending to do harm, (b) is restricted to extraordinary moral disasters, and (c) targets the principle of discrimination, which prohibits intentionally harming innocents, rather than the principle of proportionality.

The first of these differences is the most easily dealt with. In just war theory the threat is antagonistic. There is an unjust aggressor who threatens harm to innocents. In the context of many other emergencies where we might seek to justify surveillance, such as the Coronavirus pandemic, the threat will be non-antagonistic. There may be persons who act irresponsibly, e.g., by failing to take reasonable precautions to avoid infecting others, but many emergencies will involve people who intentionally harm others, if at all, only as fringe cases. A pathogen, for example, is only metaphorically speaking an antagonist.

It is difficult to see, however, why the difference in the type of threat should affect whether the state of emergency creates a moral exception. The moral exception is supposedly a result of the magnitude of the harm threatened, not of the specific nature of the harm. Thus, it would seem strange to say that a moral constraint is relaxed or overridden in the case where enormous harm is threatened by attack from an unjust military attack, so that we can permissibly act to avert the threat in ways that would ordinarily be impermissible, but that the same is not true for situations where an equal threat is posed by e.g., a natural disaster (cf. Sandin 2009).

Consider next the necessary scale of the moral disaster. A supreme emergency must be understood in reference to a 'typical emergency'. In the just war context, states or adversaries are already engaged in active, military conflict. A supreme emergency is a situation above and beyond the normal horrors of war. Walzer claims that a supreme emergency arises only when a community faces a threat that is both imminent and extreme. His illustration is the threat of Nazi invasion and occupation of the British Isles during the Second World War, i.e., replacement of

---

[3] For critical responses, see (Orend 2005; Primoratz 2011; Sandin 2009; Schwenkenbecher 2009; Statman 2012; Toner 2005). For the purposes of the present discussion, only certain issues from the debate within just war ethics are pertinent. I reference these as they arise.

the UK's liberal-democratic institutions with genocidal fascist tyranny. This is important, because if the bar for exceptional circumstances is set this high, then it will rarely be met. And when it is not, the standard *jus in bello* constraints apply.

Can the scale of emergencies where we contemplate the proportionality of surveillance rise to such extreme levels? It seems conceivable that they can. Even if, for example, the 2020–1 Coronavirus pandemic does not qualify, there is presumably *some* point where the infection mortality rate of a disease becomes high enough that a pandemic would constitute a supreme emergency. The global infection mortality rate for the Coronavirus pandemic has been estimated as *c.*0.7 per cent (Meyerowitz-Katz and Merone 2020). Plausibly, a pandemic with the *c.*50 per cent case mortality rate of Ebola would be more than sufficiently bad to qualify[4] (Shultz et al. 2016). Thus, it seems indisputable that a pandemic, or another situation that calls for surveillance, is *in principle* capable of constituting an emergency of the required magnitude.[5]

Finally, the most important of the three differences is that the moral exception in just war theory targets the principle of discrimination, which is an (otherwise) absolute constraint on intentionally harming innocents. The central argument for the supreme emergency exemption is the counterintuitive implications of sustaining this constraint in the face of a supreme emergency. Many find the *fiat justitia ruat caelum*[6] spirit of the absolute constraint implausible, when the price of respecting it is a moral disaster on the scale of e.g., genocide or societal collapse.

Proponents of the qualitative difference view can plausibly argue, however, that this difference is not decisive. First and foremost because one plausible modern interpretation of the principle of discrimination is that it is a result of the liability weights attached to individual welfare in our proportionality evaluation (McMahan 2004). On this interpretation, the reason why it is wrong to attack innocents is that because they are not liable to attack, harming them counts dramatically more in our proportionality assessment. To those who resist this interpretation of the principle of discrimination, the proponent can further point out that it is plausible that a situation which dramatically affects one constraint on our actions will also affect other constraints when similar moral factors are at stake. Thus, if we can override the principle of discrimination *because* the magnitude of harm threatened has exceeded a threshold, might it not also be the case that we can reduce the required ratio for proportionality *because* the magnitude of harm has exceeded the threshold?

---

[4] One should bear in mind, of course, the difference between infection mortality rates and case mortality rates. The point stands, however, for any realistic relation between the two.

[5] Determining whether the Coronavirus pandemic is or is not a threat of sufficient magnitude is inhibited by the fact that the required magnitude is woefully underspecified in the literature on supreme emergency exemptions (Schwenkenbecher 2009). It is not clear, that is, exactly where to set the threshold, or why the threshold must be set precisely there. I return to this point briefly below.

[6] Traditionally translated as 'Let justice be done though the heavens fall.'

## Against the Qualitative Difference View

In the above I have set out the qualitative difference view and sketched some possible motivations. It is, I hope to have shown, both a coherent view, and a view with some minimal plausibility due to its similarity to views that have been defended in the literature. Nonetheless, in this section, I will argue that the view is vulnerable to such serious objections that we should reject it. We must look instead to the quantitative difference view, which I sketch in the next section.

The most obvious objection to the qualitative difference view is that it implausibly entails that situations that differ only to the smallest possible extent in the magnitude of the threat can nonetheless differ enormously in how we ought to morally assess them.[7] This charge of moral alchemy is a well-established challenge for threshold views in ethics, but it seems to me particularly egregious in the present case (cf. Alexander 2000). We can illustrate the problem as follows: suppose we define, purely for the purposes of illustration, constant $k_1$ as 2:1, constant $k_2$ as 3:2, and the threshold T as 100. Now, consider:

**Three scenarios.**  In scenario 1, public health surveillance ($\phi_1$) would avert a public health threat of magnitude 90, at a surveillance cost of 60. In scenario 2, public health surveillance ($\phi_2$) would avert a public health threat of magnitude 99 at a surveillance cost of 50. In scenario 3, public health surveillance ($\phi_3$) would avert a public health threat of magnitude 100, at a surveillance cost of 66.

The comparative proportionality assessments in *three scenarios* are very counterintuitive:

> $\varphi_1$ is disproportional, because it is below the threshold and the ratio of goods over bads is less than 2:1 (90:60 = 3:2).

> $\varphi_2$ is also disproportional, because it is below the threshold and the ratio of goods over bads is less than 2:1 (99:50).

> $\varphi_3$ is proportional, because it is above the threshold, and the ratio of goods is equal to or greater than 3:2 (100:66 ≈ 3:2).

One way of illustrating how counterintuitive the comparative proportionality assessments are, is to imagine the complaints that the persons harmed by the unaverted health threat in scenario 2 might reasonably make. The ratio of goods over bads produced by surveillance in their scenario would have been substantially better than the ratio in scenario 3. In fact, the ratio in scenario 3 is on a par with

---

[7] Statman discusses a version of this problem as 'the continuum problem' (Statman 2012).

scenario 1. And yet, the great increase in the ratio of scenario 2 relative to scenario 1 makes no difference to the permissibility of surveillance in scenario 2, in spite of the fact that the proportionality condition is supposed to be grounded in and sensitive to this exact consideration. On the other hand, the single step in scenario 3 from a threat of magnitude 99 to one of magnitude 100 was sufficient to make surveillance proportional, in spite of the fact that the ratio of goods over bads in scenario 3 is dramatically worse than in scenario 2.[8] As for the change in the magnitude of the threat that generates the moral exception, the change in threat from scenario 1 to scenario 2 is *nine* times as great as the change from scenario 2 to scenario 3, and yet again the former change made no difference to the moral permissibility of health surveillance in scenario 2. Surely, the persons harmed in scenario 2 might say, it is absurd that they were denied protection on the above basis?

A second challenge for the qualitative difference view closely related to the first is that it makes our moral assessment implausibly sensitive to how we individuate threats and acts of surveillance.[9] Consider first how we might individuate threats. We might speak e.g., of the Coronavirus pandemic as one threat, but very often threats of the relevant magnitude will be equally (or more) plausibly conceived of as a series of related threats, e.g., the millions of spatially and temporally distributed infections with Coronavirus that jointly constitute a pandemic. If we require threats to be single events, e.g., the impact of a very large asteroid on Earth, then the qualitative difference view will not apply to most of the events that its proponents presumably would want to apply it to. So proponents will likely favour the aggregative view of threats, where separate events can jointly constitute a threat that surpasses T. This raises immediate difficulties however. Suppose again that we define constant $k_1$ as 2:1, constant $k_2$ as 3:2, and the threshold T as 100. Now consider:

**Distributed threats:**   Threat A is a pandemic composed of millions of individual infections, which can be prevented by a programme of health surveillance, $\phi_1$. In aggregate, averting threat A is a good of 100, equalling threshold T, and the ratio of goods over bads is 3:2, equalling the required proportionality ratio at or above T. Threats B and C, on the other hand, are single, separate events, each of which

[8] Note that the problem here isn't, as in the Sorites paradox, that regardless of where we define the threshold, it sounds strange to say that there is a sharp distinction between cases just on each side of the line (Hyde and Raffman 2018). That difficulty, if it is one, afflicts both the quantitative and qualitative views of proportionality. The problem here is that the very same considerations that count in favour of permissibility can make no difference when they occur on one side of the line, and all the difference when they occur on the other, even when the former are stronger than the latter. And unlike Sorites, where one horn of the dilemma is the absurdity of insisting, e.g., that all (or no) men are bald, the quantitative view, which avoids this difficulty, is not inherently implausible.
[9] (Statman 2012) makes a similar argument.

can be prevented by surveillance programme $\phi_2$. Averting threats B and C are each goods of 75, while the proportionality ratio of $\phi_2$ for each threat is 15:8.

Note first that individually considered, averting the infections of threat A would be disproportional, since 3:2 is below the proportionality ratio for threats below T. Only jointly do the infections constitute a threat of magnitude T. Note also that threats B and C would jointly constitute a threat of even greater magnitude (150). Nonetheless, the single programme ($\phi_2$), that would avert both of them is disproportional, this despite the fact that the total good it does is much greater (150 vs. 100) and the proportionality ratio more favourable (15:8 vs. 3:2). This is implausible. At the very least, the onus is on the proponent of the qualitative difference view to at once establish how we distinguish the threats that can and should be aggregated from the threats that should not, and to explain why the suggested way of separating threats justifies such radically different moral assessments of the surveillance programmes that could avert them.

Similar problems arise for individuating actions. In the above, I have assumed that we can meaningfully speak of, e.g., a health surveillance programme as one action, whose proportionality can be assessed. But very often, surveillance will in fact be equally (or more) plausibly conceived as a set of related actions, potentially millions or billions of individual acts of data-collection that feed into a single database. How are we to assess the proportionality of such actions? If we assess them individually, then again, we are unlikely to find many examples of actions that meet threshold T. It is rare indeed, for a single act to be capable of preventing bads on the scale at stake in exceptional circumstances. More likely, the proponent of the qualitative difference view will hold, as above with threats, that actions can be part of an action set, and that proportionality can be assessed for the action set as a whole.

A first issue with aggregating acts is that there will be cases similar to *distributed threats*, where we must counterintuitively hold certain actions to be disproportional although they do more good relative to bad than other actions that are proportional, simply because the latter are, and the former are not, part of an action set that jointly averts a threat of at least magnitude T. As with the individuation of threats, the proponent of the qualitative view must both develop an account of how to distinguish actions that should be assessed in aggregate from those that should not and explain why proportionality is different in the two cases. And as with the individuation of threats, it is difficult to see what a plausible such account could look like.

In addition, the aggregation of actions raises a further problem. The problem is that this can force us to say that acts that are individually grossly disproportional are nonetheless both permissible and proportional, simply because they are part of the relevant action set. Suppose as before that $k_1$ is 2:1, $k_2$ is 3:2, and T is 100. Consider:

*Curate's egg.*   $\phi_1$ and $\phi_2$ are individual acts of surveillance to help mitigate a public health emergency that jointly constitute an action set. $\phi_1$ brings about 90 good at a surveillance cost of 45. $\phi_2$ brings about 10 good at a surveillance cost of 10.

Jointly, the action set is proportional *because* the addition of $\phi_2$ brings the set above T (100:55 $\geq$ 3:2, but not 2:1). Individually considered, however, $\phi_1$ is proportional (90:45 $\geq$ 2:1), while $\phi_2$ is grossly disproportional (10:10 $\ll$ 2:1). $\phi_2$ becomes permissible only as part of the action set. The quantitative difference view avoids this problem, since it can simply apply the proportionality condition to each individual act, and consistently hold that acts either are or are not proportional (cf. Alexander 2000: 899–900). In a slogan, the qualitative difference view requires us to evaluate proportionality on average, while the quantitative difference view allows us to evaluate proportionality at the margin.

The qualitative difference view, I suggested, is not immediately implausible. However, on consideration, we can see that it faces very serious difficulties in the shape of strongly counterintuitive implications. It is implausible that very small differences in the stakes of a threat can make dramatic differences to the proportionality of actions that avert the threat, that we can aggregate threats and actions such that the aggregated threats and actions are subject to different proportionality considerations, and that aggregation allows individually disproportional actions to become proportional.[10] In sum, I take it that these difficulties should lead us to reject the qualitative difference view.

## An Unexceptional Theory of Proportional Surveillance

I have argued above that we ought to reject the qualitative difference view. This leaves us with the quantitative difference view, and what we may earnestly call an unexceptional theory of proportional surveillance. In this section, I sketch such an unexceptional proportionality condition for morally permissible surveillance in exceptional circumstances. I also briefly discuss which values to measure and compare, arguing that some of the most obvious goods and bads are at least in principle comparable.

There are different ways of conceiving of an unexceptional proportionality condition (Henschke 2018). Perhaps the simplest plausible account of a proportionality condition for morally permissible surveillance is the teleological account (Thomsen 2020). On **the teleological account**:

---

[10] Some might add that the qualitative view presupposes a non-arbitrary way of specifying $T$. The general difficulty of specifying deontological thresholds is both obvious and well recognized in the literature (Alexander 2000: 905–10; Ellis 1992). However, it is not clear to me that this difficulty constitutes a challenge to the plausibility as opposed to the implementation of threshold views (Arneson 2018).

An act φ of surveillance is proportional in the sense relevant to moral permissibility *iff* the goods that φ'ing brings about are equal to or greater than the bads that φ'ing brings about.

Let me clarify three features of the teleological account as a quantitative view.

First, the goods and bads φ'ing brings about should be measured, I believe, relative to a counterfactual baseline defined by the goods and bads brought about in each of the relevant action alternatives. It is a point of contention, however, what the relevant action alternatives are for any given act of surveillance. The alternative of *not* carrying out surveillance can be included, in which case the (wide) proportionality consideration makes a separate necessity condition redundant (Lazar 2017). Uncontroversially, alternative ways of carrying out the surveillance should also be included, as should alternatives to surveillance that bring about the same goods. There are further persuasive arguments to the effect that action alternatives that bring about *similar* goods must also be included (Oberman 2019). As one extends the scope for alternatives that bring about similar goods, however, proportionality becomes steadily more demanding. Eventually, without some restriction of scope, the proportionality condition collapses into the necessity condition of consequentialism: that an action is morally permissible only if it has consequences at least as good as those of any alternative action available (but not, of course, the consequentialist sufficiency claim, that an action *is* morally permissible if it has such consequences).

Second, the teleological account is by definition incompatible with the qualitative difference view, because the qualitative difference view requires that $k_1$ is greater than 1:1, on pain of allowing that acts above T can permissibly avert disaster even though they bring about even worse outcomes (because $k_2$ is smaller than $k_1$ and therefore smaller than 1:1). This constitutes at best a weak reason to doubt the qualitative difference view, however, since proponents of the qualitative difference view can simply interpret the incompatibility as evidence against the teleological account (one person's *modus ponens* is another's *modus tollens*). We should reject the qualitative view for other reasons, as discussed above.

Third, it is worth noting that a quantitative difference view can be both more restrictive and more permissive than a qualitative difference view. This depends entirely on how the required ratios of each of the views are defined. If the alternatives are a quantitative difference view which defines $k_1$ as 2:1, and a qualitative difference view which defines $k_1$ as 2:1 and $k_2$ as 3:2, then the qualitative difference view will be identical to the quantitative difference view below the threshold, but more permissive above it. This is the most common idea of the relation between the two views. It is not the only possible relation, however. To take just one example, if the qualitative difference view instead defines $k_1$ as 3:1 and $k_2$ as 2:1, then the qualitative difference view will be more demanding below the threshold and as permissive as the quantitative view above it.

We have postponed until now a more focused look at the goods and bads of surveillance. The goods of surveillance will often be relatively well defined. Surveillance that averts or mitigates a global pandemic, for example, brings about goods in the shape of better health. Health is uncontroversially valuable as a constitutive of well-being. It is also quantifiable and measurable as QALY's[11] (McKie, Richardson, Singer, and Kuhse 1998; Williams 1995) In addition to health, surveillance that averts or mitigates an emergency might bring about economic goods (e.g., preventing economic losses), social goods (e.g., ensuring the continued ability to enjoy social events), and psychological goods (e.g., avoiding fear, sorrow, and anxiety). These goods are plausibly valuable because they are constituents of or contribute to well-being, and as such, at least in theory, comparable.

The bads of surveillance generally, and public health surveillance specifically, are less well defined. In a recent, short article, Morley et al. suggest that public health surveillance 'may exacerbate problems like social panic, social shaming, the erosion of trust in the government and public health services, or inequality. Furthermore, it may facilitate potentially unethical uses of personal data originally collected for the purpose of contact tracing that may impact privacy, severely and perhaps irreversibly' (Morley et al. 2020: 3). Alan Rubel adds the plausible suggestion that '[t]he possibility of having their health information disclosed may lead to people avoiding care, which is generally detrimental to their health and hence interests regardless of their particular conceptions of the good' (Rubel 2012: 13). These concerns track plausible bads that have also been recognized in the broader surveillance literature (e.g., Macnish 2015; Solove 2006, 2007). Conveniently, they are also bads whose disvalue can ultimately, like the goods above, be grounded in well-being. This is an advantage, since it ensures commensurability—we will be able to compare goods and bads when weighing proportionality.

## Conclusion

In a time of emergency, it may be tempting to believe that the constraints on our behaviour, which apply in ordinary circumstances, should no longer bind us. In the face of catastrophe, we may need to resort to radical measures that would in other cases be morally impermissible. Or so the thinking might go.

In this chapter, I hope to have argued persuasively that at least one version of such views—the qualitative difference view of proportionality in surveillance—is implausible. Whatever we take the proportionality condition relevant to morally

---

[11] The use of QALYs in healthcare policy is controversial. However, the most important controversies concern the use of utilitarianism as the theory of priority-setting, as opposed to. e.g. theories sensitive to fairness in distribution of goods.

permissible surveillance to be, it applies equally to ordinary circumstances and exceptional circumstances.

One plausible interpretation of the push towards the qualitative difference view is that it is motivated by the combination of a sense of urgency in the face of dramatic or potentially catastrophic circumstances, and an awareness of the difficulty of performing the conventional proportionality evaluation. Not only are many of the empirical factors that go into the equation uncertain and very difficult to clarify, but our theory of proportional surveillance is itself much less developed than one might have hoped. A natural response to these facts is that we cannot afford to expend time and efforts attempting, perhaps in vain, to work out what level of surveillance would be proportional. This sentiment might make the qualitative difference view appear attractive. If the qualitative difference view were true, then there is less reason to do so. The qualitative difference view *justifies* our favoured response, of leaving proportionality evaluations for situations where we can better afford to explore it at our leisure.

There is a kernel of insight in this line of thinking. The kernel is this: it is a very serious problem, given the enormous and growing amount of surveillance being conducted, that we do not have a consensus theory of proportional surveillance that allows us to say with *confidence* and *precision* whether a given practice of surveillance is or is not proportional in the sense relevant to moral permissibility. Ideally, we want a mathematical model with easily estimable input variables, which would allow us to confidently calculate an answer for at least the most ordinary situations.

Beyond that, however, we must reject the urgency motivation for adopting the qualitative difference view as wishful thinking (or, more technically, a fallacy of *argumentum ad consequentiam*). If urgency is to be a spur to action, then let it be a spur towards achieving the ideal theory we need. To take the proportionality of surveillance in exceptional circumstances seriously is to accept that we need urgently to develop a theory of morally proportional surveillance that is genuinely action-guiding.[12]

# References

7amleh—Arab Center for Social Media Advancement, Access Now, African Declaration on Internet Rights and Freedoms Coalition, AI Now, Algorithm Watch, Alternatif Bilisim,...World Wide Web Foundation. 2020. 'States' use of

---

[12] I have presented a draft version of this chapter at a 2020 seminar with the Criminal Justice research group, Roskilde University. I am grateful for comments from Sebastian Holmen, Rune Klingenberg, Ditte Marie Munch-Jurisic, Kasper Lippert-Rasmussen, Jesper Ryberg, Thomas Søbirk Petersen, and Søren Sofus Wichmann. I owe further thanks for very helpful comments to Adam Henschke.

digital surveillance technologies to fight pandemic must respect human rights'. Press release. https://freedomhouse.org/article/states-use-digital-surveillance-technologies-fight-pandemic-must-respect-human-rights.

Alexander, L. 2000. 'Deontology at the Threshold'. *San Diego Law Review* 37 (4): 893–912.

Arneson, R. 2018. 'Deontology's Travails'. In *Moral Puzzles and Legal Perplexities: Essays on the Influence of Larry Alexander*, edited by H. M. Hurd, 350–70. Cambridge: Cambridge University Press.

Bamford, R., H. Dace, B. Macon-Cooney, C. and Yiu. 2020. *A Price Worth Paying: Tech, Privacy and the Fight Against Covid-19*. https://institute.global/policy/price-worth-paying-tech-privacy-and-fight-against-covid-19.

Brown, I. and D. Korff. 2009. 'Terrorism and the Proportionality of Internet Surveillance'. *European Journal of Criminology* 6 (2): 119–34. doi:10.1177/1477370808100541.

Ellis, A. 1992. 'Deontology, Incommensurability and the Arbitrary'. *Philosophy and Phenomenological Research* 52 (4): 855–75. doi:10.2307/2107914.

Ferretti, L., C. Wymant, M. Kendall, L. Zhao, A. Nurtay, A., L. Abeler-Dörner et al. 2020. 'Quantifying SARS-CoV-2 Transmission Suggests Epidemic Control with Digital Contact Tracing'. *Science* 368 (6491). doi:10.1126/science.abb6936.

Heller, J. 2020. 'Israel Imposes Cyber-Monitoring of Coronavirus Cases'. *Reuters*, 17 March. https://www.reuters.com/article/health-coronavirus-israel-idUSL8N2BA2DH.

Henschke, A. 2018. 'Are the Costs of Metadata Worth It? Conceptualising Proportionality and Its Relation to Metadata'. In *Intelligence and the Function of Government*, edited by D. Baldino and R. Crawley. Carlton: Melbourne University Press.

Hyde, D. and D. Raffman. 2018. 'Sorites Paradox'. In *The Stanford Encyclopedia of Philosophy*, edited by E. N. Zalta.

Kagan, S. 1988. *Normative Ethics*. Boulder: Westview Press.

Kant, I. 1797. 'Über ein vermeintes Recht aus Menschenliebe zu lügen'. In:

Kant, I. 1993. 'On a Supposed Right to Lie because of Philanthropic Concerns'. In *Grounding for the Metaphysics of Morals*, edited by J. W. Ellington. Indianapolis: Hackett.

Lazar, S. 2017. 'War'. In *The Stanford Encyclopedia of Philosophy*, edited by E. N. Zalta.

Macnish, K. 2015. 'An Eye for an Eye: Proportionality and Surveillance'. *Ethical Theory and Moral Practice* 18 (3): 529–48.

Macnish, K. 2018. 'Government Surveillance and Why Defining Privacy Matters in a Post-Snowden World'. *Journal of Applied Philosophy* 35 (2): 417–32.

McKie, J., J. Richardson, P. Singer, and H. Kuhse, H. 1998. *The Allocation of Health Care Resources: An Ethical Evaluation of the 'QALY' Approach*. Farnham: Ashgate.

McMahan, J. 2004. 'The Ethics of Killing in War'. *Ethics* 114: 693–733.

Meyerowitz-Katz, G. and L. Merone. 2020. 'A Systematic Review and Meta-Analysis of Published Research Data on COVID-19 Infection-Fatality Rates'. *International Journal of Infectious Diseases*. doi:10.1016/j.ijid.2020.09.1464.

Morley, J., J. Cowls, M. Taddeo, and L. Floridi. 2020. 'Ethical Guidelines for SARS-CoV-2 Digital Tracking and Tracing Systems'. In. Oxford: Oxford Internet Institute. https://papers.ssrn.com/sol3/papers.cfm?abstract_id=3582550

O, C. 2020. 'StopCovid ou encore?' *Medium*, 3 May. https://cedric-o.medium.com/stopcovid-ou-encore-b5794d99bb12.

Oberman, K. 2019. 'War and Poverty'. *Philosophical Studies*, 176 (1): 197–217.

Orend, B. 2005. 'Is there a Supreme Emergency Exemption?' In *Just War Theory*, edited by M. Evans, 134–55. New York: Palgrave Macmillan.

Primoratz, I. 2011. 'Civilian Immunity, Supreme Emergency, and Moral Disaster'. *The Journal of Ethics* 15 (4): 371–86.

Rubel, A. 2012. 'Justifying Public Health Surveillance: Basic Interests, Unreasonable Exercise, and Privacy'. *Kennedy Institute of Ethics Journal* 22 (1): 1–33.

Rønn, K. V. and K. Lippert-Rasmussen. 2020. 'Out of Proportion? On Surveillance and the Proportionality Requirement'. *Ethical Theory Moral Practice*. Online first. doi:10.1007/s10677-019-10057-z.

Sandin, P. 2009. 'Supreme Emergencies without the Bad Guys'. *Philosophia* 37 (1): 153–67.

Schwenkenbecher, A. 2009. 'Terrorism, Supreme Emergency and Killing the Innocent. *Perspectives—The Review of International Affairs* 17 (1): 105–26.

Shultz, J. M., Z. Espinel, M. Espinola, and A. Rechkemmer. 2016. 'Distinguishing Epidemiological Features of the 2013–2016 West Africa Ebola Virus Disease Outbreak'. *Disaster Health* 3 (3): 78–88. doi:10.1080/21665044.2016.1228326.

Singer, N., and Sang-Hun, C. 2020. 'As Coronavirus Surveillance Escalates, Personal Privacy Plummets'. *New York Times*. https://www.nytimes.com/2020/03/23/technology/coronavirus-surveillance-tracking-privacy.html?auth=login-google&login=email

Solove, D. J. 2006. A Taxonomy of Privacy. *University of Pennsylvania Law Review* 154 (3): 477–560.

Solove, D. J. 2007. '"I've Got Nothing to Hide" and Other Misunderstandings of Privacy'. *San Diego Law Review* 44: 745–72.

Stanley, J. and J. S. Granick. 2020. *The Limits of Location Tracking in an Epidemic*. Retrieved from https://www.aclu.org/sites/default/files/field_document/limits_of_location_tracking_in_an_epidemic.pdf

Statman, D. 2012. 'Supreme Emergencies and the Continuum Problem'. *Journal of Military Ethics* 11 (4): 287–98.

Tele-2/Watson, 2016. https://eur-lex.europa.eu/legal-content/EN/TXT/?uri=CELEX%3A62015CJ0203

The European Commission. 2020. 'Commission Recommendation (EU) 2020/518'. Press release.

Thomsen, F. K. 2020. 'The Teleological Account of Proportional Surveillance'. *Res Publica* 26: 373–401. doi:https://doi.org/10.1007/s11158-020-09451-7

Toner, C. 2005. 'Just War and the Supreme Emergency Exemption'. *Philosophical Quarterly* 55 (221): 545–61.

Walzer, M. 1977. *Just and Unjust Wars* (Vol. 92). New York: Basic Books.

Williams, A. 1995. 'Economics, QALYs and Medical Ethics—a Health Economist's Perspective'. *Health Care Analysis* 3 (3): 221–6. doi:10.1007/BF02197671.

# 12

# Technofixing Surveillance

## A Proportionate Response?

*Kevin Macnish*

In times of crisis, people, not unreasonably, expect something to be done. Those in charge look to meet the needs of and present the favoured solution to the population, where it is digested and accepted or rejected. In a health crisis in which a virus is spreading rapidly, with often fatal implications, surveillance of the virus's progress becomes central to a government's understanding of the scale of the problem and the efficacy of its solutions. In such cases, there is clearly a justified cause for surveillance (Macnish 2014). However, while surveillance per se may be justified, it does not follow that *all* surveillance may be justified. Some acts of surveillance may be excessively intrusive or indiscriminate. To put it in terms of a just surveillance framework, there may be a *jus ad speculando*, but the *jus in specluandum* remains to be determined (Macnish 2014).

Responses to crises are often sought in technology, be that health, finance, war, or elsewhere. This in itself is not surprising. Technology, on the whole, exists to solve our problems (or, more cynically, to solve problems that we didn't know we had until the technology was invented). It seems reasonable to turn to 'the latest methods' to respond to the crisis, be that punch cards, computers, mobile phones, or implanted chips. This may come at the risk of ignoring older methods which have worked in the past to a limited degree. Surely the new technology can deal with the problem faster, and more accurately? I am not the first to refer to this perspective as 'techno-fetishism' (Beier 2006, 2003; Pomarède 2018; Tierney 1992: 90).

In this chapter I argue that these two concerns: the urge to respond to a crisis and the readiness to seek a solution in technology (a 'technofix') lead to the introduction of ethically disproportionate responses. This might seem curious in light of the first concern, the urge to do something, often being portrayed itself as a carefully thought-out and proportionate response to the crisis. My argument is that a lack of imagination and public discussion, coupled with techno-fetishism, leads to less or non-technical yet preferable responses being overlooked.

The argument takes as its prime illustration the track and trace apps (TTAs) developed in Europe and the US on the basis of code developed jointly by Apple and Google (the AGTTA) in response to the Covid-19 virus (Li and Guo

Kevin Macnish, *Technofixing Surveillance: A Proportionate Response?* In: *The Ethics of Surveillance in Times of Emergency.*
Edited by: Kevin Macnish and Adam Henschke, Oxford University Press. © Oxford University Press 2023.
DOI: 10.1093/oso/9780192864918.003.0013

2020; Sharon 2020). While this demonstrates the case, the argument itself is far wider and can be seen in other historical cases. I refer to these through the chapter where pertinent.

I begin with a brief discussion of proportionality, drawing on Henschke's analysis of the concept (Henschke 2018). This analysis demonstrates that there are different ways of understanding and using the term, which leads to confusion in the public debate. I then describe the technology behind AGTTA and how this may lead to false positive and false negatives. This leads into a discussion on the ethical harms which may arise from the use of the AGTTA technology. I then return to Henschke's analysis to demonstrate how the AGTTA technology may be seen as proportionate in the light of one approach and yet disproportionate in the light of alternative approaches. I suggest that these alternatives are often not presented to the public debate owing to the aforementioned tendency to techno-fetishism. As such, I conclude that the form of surveillance undertaken by AGTTA and other technofixes, careful as they may be, may nonetheless be disproportion-ate responses to the crises they seek to address.

## Proportionality

Proportionality has long been considered a pertinent ethical concern with regards to surveillance, although its precise determination is not straightforward. Considerations of proportionality as an element of moral philosophy date to the Nicomachean Ethics (2004, bk. V), and further in religious literature to 'life for life, eye for eye' (Exodus 21:23). In the last 30 years proportionality has been posited as a central component in the ethics of surveillance (Macnish 2015), intelligence (Bellaby 2014; Omand 2012; Quinlan 2007), self-defence (Uniacke 2011), jurispru-dential sentencing (Slobogin 1998), and war (Cavanaugh 2006; Hurka 2005; Kamm 1991; Quinn 1989). Appeal has also been made to proportionality in writings on the environment (Steel 2013; Turner 2013), income distribution (Cappelen and Tungodden 2017), investor interests (Krommendijk and Morijn 2009), animal welfare (Cheyne and Alder 2007), and computing (Iachello and Abowd 2005).

Proportionality has also been a key consideration in laws regulating surveil-lance. In the UK, the Investigatory Powers Act (IPA 2016) requires acts of surveillance to be necessary and proportionate (Section 61 (1c)). In the US, the Supreme Court discussed in Terry vs Ohio (392 U.S. 1 (1968)) whether stop and search, within the context of the Fourth Amendment forbidding arbitrary search and seizure, merited a proportionate justification (see the discussion in Slobogin 1998: 1066–70). In Europe, proportionality is a central consideration for surveil-lance practices and counterterrorism actions (De Hert 2005; Michaelsen 2010).

Within analytic philosophy, proportionality has less of a history, with some notable exceptions such as Jeff McMahan's *Killing in War* (2011) and Thomas

Hurka's *Proportionality in the Morality of War* (2005), from which my paper *Eye for an Eye: Proportionality and Surveillance* (2015) draws to clarify the role of proportionality in surveillance practice. More recently, papers on surveillance and proportionality have been published by Thomsen (2020), Rønn and Lippert-Rasmussen (2020), and the aforementioned work by Henschke (2018).

Henschke's paper is of particular note to the present discussion. He identifies five approaches in which the concept proportionality is employed. These include appropriateness, the means used contrasted with the end sought (e.g., using armed police to break up a peaceful demonstration); action versus inaction, contrasting the act in question with not acting (e.g., not using armed police to break up the demonstration); comparing costs and benefits (e.g., the harms of using armed police against the costs of not using them); comparing alternative means to achieving a desired end (e.g., using armed police compared with surveillance drones); and comparing simple with complex acts such that an apparently simple act (e.g., using armed police to break up a peaceful demonstration) may be excessive, but a more complex description (e.g., using armed police to break up a peaceful demonstration under the cover of which a terrorist is trying to gain proximity to kill a politician) may be more subtle.

Building on Henschke's analysis, there are two approaches to proportionality of especial pertinence to the current chapter. The first, the fear of not using TTAs as a technofix to the problem of infection, draws on Henschke's second approach of action versus inaction. If the population does not use the app then people will die and, while there may be harms, these are outweighed by the benefits of its use. This contrasts a society faced with using the TTA or not using the TTA and, in the latter case, having nothing with which to replace it. This is the argument taken in public debate to justify the use of AGTTA in the case of Covid-19 and other technologies in the past.

The second approach is that of comparing alternative means to achieving a desired end. In this case, technofixes are compared with non-technological (or older technological) approaches to determine which is the 'best' means to achieve the desired end (i.e., tracking and tracing of people who are at heightened risk of infection from the virus). For reasons I discuss in the following section, 'best' in this case means not only the most effective, but the most effective which also has the most ethical impact (in terms of minimizing harm while achieving good and respecting fundamental rights, not least individual privacy). This was the techno-fix sought by AGTTA over other solutions employed in countries such as South Korea and China (Kostka and Habich-Sobiegalla 2020; Li and Guo 2020; Ryan 2020). However, while the AGTTA solution may have been less ethically harmful than alternative TTAs, I will argue that alternatives to technofixes rarely enter the debate. The silence on the part of less or non-technical alternatives means that these approaches are frequently overlooked such that more ethically proportionate responses may be ignored.

## Efficacy of Technology

New technologies, especially when introduced in a crisis, are often sold as pana-ceas to a problem (Esposito et al. 2018; Gazendam and Kerkhoff 1999; Singh and Thomas 2019; R. D. Williams 2001). It is rarely the case, though, that they genuinely solve the problem at hand. Not only do they frequently fail to resolve the problem *in toto*, but they also introduce new problems and rarely function as well as is claimed (Huesemann and Huesemann 2011; Johnston 2020; Wells 2008). This has been well demonstrated by the plethora of 'track and trace' apps (TTAs) across the world in response to Covid-19.

One of the most notable differences among TTAs has been whether they are centralized or decentralized (Raman et al. 2021). The former collect pertinent information about the user (location, proximity, duration) over time and relay this to a central database, typically operated by the state. This has the obvious advantage of a pre-existent national infrastructure and, at least in theory, a smooth integration with national healthcare responses. Such an approach to TTAs has been taken in Australia, Canada, South Korea, Qatar, and Singapore (Raman et al. 2021). The negative side, at least for some, is that this places considerable information about the users into the hands of the state, particularly when that state already displays authoritarian tendencies or engages in authori-tarian activities. The TTAs allow the state security apparatus to form a clear understanding of who is meeting whom, when and where, irrespective of whether they have contracted the virus. As such, they introduce new levels of state surveillance that would be problematic, even in many contemporary authoritarian states, in normal circumstances. It remains to be seen whether the TTAs will be dismantled when the threat of the current virus recedes. However, the history of surveillance suggests that this is unlikely to be the case, with governments typically increasing surveillance capacities over time and rarely rolling the same back (Macnish 2018: 9–29).

In the global West, following a liberal democratic and citizen rights-based tradition, a more decentralized approach has been favoured to TTAs in response to Covid-19. This is precisely to counter the concerns of centralized state surveil-lance at an unprecedented level, which runs counter to liberal-democratic values. As such, a decentralized TTA has frequently been seen to be ethically preferable to the centralized alternatives discussed above. While not adopted universally, foun-dational code for a decentralized system was developed jointly by Apple and Google and made available to interested governments. This has become the default system for TTAs in Europe and the US and will be the system I presume and critique for the remainder of this chapter.

The heart of the AGTTA runs using Bluetooth technology (as opposed to more battery intensive location systems such as GPS), identifying other users of the TTA to form networks of proximity which are held in the phone's memory for a specified duration. The principle requires that everyone has the same TTA on their phone and that users keep Bluetooth operating on their phone at all times. If a user tests positive then this is entered manually into the TTA, which then informs the TTAs of other users who have been in proximity to the positive user in the preceding forty-eight hours. The recipient TTAs then inform their users that they may have contracted Covid-19 and that they should therefore have a test. Until having the test, and if they test positive, then they should self-quarantine for up to fourteen days. At no point is user information returned to a central source.

While this is a good attempt at a decentralized TTA, there are clearly numerous ways in which the system can fail to work. To be fair, AGTTA was not marketed by Apple or Google as being 100 per cent reliable, but to encourage widespread adoption, governments frequently presented it as a reliable response and a worthwhile investment (Apple 2020; Burgess 2020). Nonetheless, obvious areas for the system to fail to produce the desired result can be broken down into two broad areas: human and technical. The former include, but are not limited to:

- users not carrying their phone with them;
- users having their phones turned off, or the battery flat;
- users not having Bluetooth enabled on their phone;
- users not seeking a test immediately on being informed that they may be infected;
- users not entering their positive test result into the app immediately;
- asymptomatic users not being tested and so not entering data into the app.

Technical areas of failure to produce the required result include:

- users passing within the necessary radius of an infected user, but the infected user is wearing effective PPE or behind a partition or screen which prevents transfer;
- users contracting the virus from handling infected items rather than from proximity to an infected person.

I am not making an argument here that the companies who develop TTAs are making overblown claims to perfect accuracy. Generally they do not, and they have, in the case of Covid-19 apps, stressed that this is one part of an overall response ecosystem (Apple 2020). Governments encouraging take-up of the TTA have sometimes presented it as reliable and at other times presented it, like the companies, as a part of an overall response system (Field 2020). How users hear and interpret these warnings and instructions is a different matter again. While one may argue that there is only so much that companies and the government can do to warn against false understanding, it is also important to accept that TTAs will be used by many people, many of whom will not read the full warnings and instructions (Acquisti and Grossklags 2005; Angulo et al. 2012; Nissenbaum 2011). If the app is not developed and widely marketed with this in mind, then it will be misunderstood and misused, adding to the problems in its efficacy.

The result of these problems is that use of the TTA will inevitably result in false positives and false negatives. A false positive in this case will be a TTA identifying a user as at risk of infection (although it may be interpreted as a user being infected) when that user is not at risk of infection. They may, for example, have passed within the threshold radius of an infected user, but been separated by a Perspex partition. A false negative, by contrast, fails to alert a user that they are at risk of infection (although this may be interpreted as the user not being at risk of infection) when that user in fact is at risk owing to recent proximity to an infected user. In this case, the user may have been in proximity to an asymptomatic user who has not been tested.

False positives and false negatives are ethically unproblematic when they do not lead to wrongs. There may be technical frustrations with the efficacy of the system, but this is a separate issue beyond the scope of this chapter. In the case of TTAs, though, there are harms that may or will arise through false positives and false negatives. A false positive, for example, can lead to a user fearing that they are infected, reduce their ability to work or interact with people, and an increased sense of loneliness or isolation. A false negative, by contrast, can lead to further spread of the virus, leading to death or injury and economic damage arising from self-quarantining.[1]

While false positives and negatives may be presented as relatively minor, even an error rate of 5 per cent (i.e., 95 per cent accuracy) can have significant impacts on a sizeable population. Taking the population of the UK as 70 million and assuming that 10 per cent are infected (i.e., 7 million), the error rate implies that 5 per cent of the population (3.5 million) will be informed that they are at increased risk of infection while 5 per cent of those infected (i.e., 350,000) will not be informed that they are at increased risk of infection. This leads to an overall error rate of 3.85 million, or 55 per cent of the overall infected population. This figure is then exacerbated still further by error rates in testing and people failing to self-quarantine effectively, as well as the exponential growth rate of virus transmission.

---

[1] Lest readers fear that I am placing economic damage on a par with ethical harms, my concern here is through the indirect harms of economic damage in terms of reduced government revenue leading to reduced capabilities in terms of social welfare, healthcare, and education, as well as longer term impacts on pensions. In addition, personal economic harms have significant ethical implications, such as through loss of work or reduced wages.

## Harms of Apps

I turn now to look in more detail at the harms arising from the use of decentralized TTAs. In this section I consider locational privacy, coercion and voluntariness, repeated quarantine, spread of the infection, and harms to particular (minority) communities.

Even when decentralized, TTAs risk exposing locational data of users which may reasonably be held to be private. In South Korea, where a centralized approach was used, an infection hot spot occurred in an area of Seoul known for its homosexual nightlife. Anyone found to have contracted the infection in the immediate aftermath risked being 'outed' as homosexual and might have been assumed to be inappropriately attending a nightclub and hence partying during a pandemic. In this case, locational privacy is important to protect individuals from social stigma (N. Kim 2020b). This was exacerbated in this particular case where the centralized TTA was incorporated into a nationwide 'name and shame' approach whereby people were informed not only that a neighbour might be infected, but also the name and address of that neighbour (see Sorell in this volume). While this was an instance of locational privacy lost through a centralized app, the privacy loss was not, in this case, due to that centralized nature but the confluence of an increase in infections with a location known to be a source of that increase. It is not hard to see how similar implications (and social stigmatization) can be arrived at even with decentralized systems (see, for example, fears expressed in S. N. Williams et al. 2021).

A Millean sense of autonomy as freedom to determine one's path in life has been a mainstay of post-war European and US ethics. This has only increased in the twenty-first century such that the idea of the government coercing people into downloading and using a TTA was anathema to many during the Covid-19 crisis. While rejection of even voluntary TTAs was particularly extreme in the US (where the choice to wear a face mask became politicized), even in the comparatively liberal European Union, voluntary adoption of the TTA was sparse at best. Downloads as a percentage of the population reached 35 per cent in Germany (Koptyug 2021), 17 per cent in France (Reuters 2020), and less than 10 per cent in the US (De La Garza 2020).[2] One should be cautious in comparing TTAs too directly, given that although based on the same Apple-Google designed code, each TTA had different features and requirements of users. However, when introduced to society, the apps were predicted to require a minimum saturation threshold of 60 per cent in order to function effectively (Fraser et al. 2020). Given that saturation did not come close to reaching these thresholds, one can question (a)

---

[2] Although it should be noted that as late as mid-December 2020, only nineteen US states had TTAs operating in their region (Sato 2020).

whether they are effective at all; and (b) whether they perhaps *should* be mandatory rather than voluntary if they were to work at all (Klar and Lanzerath 2020).

The third harm to arise from the use of TTAs derived from limited access to testing facilities. If the app informs the user that they are at increased risk of having contracted an infection and that user is unable (or unwilling) to be tested, then the user is expected to self-quarantine for up to fourteen days. An unwillingness to be tested may extend beyond mere intransigence to a range of issues, from active concern at the state's intentions, given that personalized test data may be collected by central government, to accessibility problems regarding test locations, which may be sparse in rural areas and oversubscribed in urban locales. The alternative of self-quarantine then takes its toll on the user who risks fear of being ill, a reduced capacity to work during the period of quarantine, a sense of loneliness and isolation, and possible stigmatization. When such alerts occur on a frequent basis then this can lead to a 'cry wolf' situation in which the alerts are eventually ignored, even when they identify genuine positives. On a nationwide scale, for those who pay attention to repeated alerts, the continued self-quarantine of individuals may also lead to significant economic issues, with knock-on effects on social welfare provision, including funding for healthcare and education.

The fourth and final set of harms to be considered here are those specifically relating to minority communities, particularly those of recent immigrants who may not have strong language skills in the nation and who may fear repression by the state. As such, the TTA may be incomprehensible to some (on grounds of language) or present itself as not being 'for them' if, in an attempt to overcome language barriers, the app uses images of predominantly white people using it. For those distrustful of the state (for whatever reason) there may be community-level distrust of the app as a tool of the state which would also affect its saturation. As of the time of writing the precise reasons are unknown, but Covid-19 was noted in the UK at least to have a disproportionate impact on members of minority communities (Pagliari 2020; Tapper 2020).

To the above concerns, one might (reasonably) respond that, while taking these harms seriously, they do not outweigh the benefits of saving lives through use of the app. Even without resorting to *ad hominem* presumptions about privilege, the response presumes that the TTA *will* work to save lives, a point I have already identified as problematic. Even given those problems, though, one might object: surely to save one life would be worth the widespread adoption and use of the app.

This raises classic utilitarian dilemmas regarding the comparative weighing and distribution of harms (such that one may question whether a hundred people being mildly injured is better or worse than one person being killed). Even then, though, any pertinent felicific calculus would need to consider not just the saving of a single life, but also the impact on lives through the imposition of repeated quarantine on a significant percentage of the population. This to be weighed against the risk of the continued spread of the virus leading to death, severe illness, or mild illness throughout the population in the absence of effective quarantine.

A natural response here might be to argue that at least TTAs in the above example identify 45 per cent of users accurately, and this is better than nothing. Better that 3.5 million people self-quarantine unnecessarily than that the infection spreads further and kills more people. To return to Henschke's analysis at the start of this chapter, this is a case of presenting the as harms a particular course of action which is proportionate to the benefits that course of action brings. Within a limited set of options, presented as TTA or no-TTA, TTA is a proportionate response.

## Alternatives

I have stressed throughout this chapter that the above presentation is an artificial dichotomy. It ignores the differences between TTAs such as those between centralized and decentralized alternatives. Here, though, the AGTTA once more appears to be the more proportionate solution in providing benefits while limiting harms through central state surveillance of the population. Admittedly, the direct benefits in terms of decreasing transmissions are, as noted above, lesser than those of the centralized model, but in liberal democracies at least, these reduced benefits may be seen to be a cost worth paying to retain core civil liberties. In this case, AGTTA comes out again as being the most proportionate response to the crisis.

There is one further step to take, though. While AGTTA may be the most proportionate *technofix* to the crisis, it does not follow that it is the most proportionate *response* to the crisis. The choice is not between a technofix and nothing, but between a technofix and non-technical solutions. The latter, I believe, are frequently ignored owing to a level of techno-fetishism in (the leadership of) society.

While there may be any number of alternative approaches to technological track and trace, for considerations of space and demonstration of the argument, I will here focus on one: local, interpersonal track and trace. In this scenario, which may occur in a pre- (or indeed post-) technological society, local resources in the form of reliable individuals (nurses, teachers, police, the military, others) are equipped with personal protective equipment and training. These people ('testers') then go door to door on a daily basis to speak to people and monitor their general health (e.g., taking temperatures, asking about recent activity, etc.). In a reasonably hierarchical system, any travel outside the area of the tester can be referred up to a supervisor so that any potential contact can be monitored. At no point will there be a need for central government to know of individuals who are infected, and yet aggregated statistics can be passed up for accurate reflections of national levels of infection.

While this approach may seem resource heavy, it should be compared with what remains an unknown expenditure on the TTAs. Furthermore, as automated responses, TTAs remove human interaction from users who may be infected, leading to the aforementioned harm of isolation and loneliness. A tester, as suggested here, increases human interaction and so reduces this particular harm. In addition, it should be noted that, in South Korea, such testers visited quarantining individuals twice each day during the Covid-19 pandemic, and so this is not an unrealistic alternative (Ryan 2020).

The presence of non-technical alternatives to TTAs therefore presents a new perspective on the proportionality consideration raised at the start of this chapter. While the consideration of responses to public health (or other) crises focuses on technofixes (techno-fetishism) then the most ethical of these technofixes will be favoured and presented as being ethically proportionate. Once the window of opportunity is opened to less or non-technical alternatives, though, options may appear which are more proportionate in terms of being less wronging of individuals while achieving similar or even better results.

## Conclusion

I have presumed in this chapter that there are cases in which surveillance may be justified in crises, including instances of tracking and tracing the development of some infections to limit harms to society. My argument is that, in terms of public debate at least, the discussion surrounding surveillance solutions to crises is dominated by technical solutions ('technofixes'). When compared to other technofixes, some may be more proportionate than others. This, I argued, was the case with AGTTA, which was presented as a proportionate response to the crisis both in terms of having limited ethical harms (so the benefits outweighed the harms) and in terms of comparison with other TTAs, such as the centralized apps used elsewhere which may have been more effective in terms of track and trace, but came at an unacceptably high ethical cost. It is hence reasonable to see AGTTA as a proportionate solution to the crisis.

However, given that all TTAs fall under the category of technofixes, I argued that non-technical solutions were subject to considerably less discussion in the public sphere. As such, it is at least plausible that while AGTTA was the most proportionate TTA, it was not the most proportionate response. The fact remains that it did risk ethical harms and, given limitations imposed by ethical concerns, was of limited efficacy.

My conclusion is not therefore that AGTTA was wrong or even that it was not proportionate. By at least one reckoning it clearly was more proportionate than alternative technofixes. It is plausible that it was also more proportionate than non-technical solutions. However, this latter point was not widely discussed in the public sphere, owing to levels of techno-fetishism in society in general and among those in positions of leadership. Until this is resolved, we risk imposing unnecessary risks on society as a result of our limited imagination, shaped by visions of technological utopias.

# References

Acquisti, A., and J. Grossklags. 2005. 'Privacy and Rationality in Individual Decision Making'. *IEEE Security Privacy* 3 (1): 26–33. https://doi.org/10.1109/MSP.2005.22.

Angulo, Julio, Simone Fischer-Hübner, Erik Wästlund, and Tobias Pulls. 2012. 'Towards Usable Privacy Policy Display and Management'. *Information Management & Computer Security*.

Apple, Google. 2020. 'Exposure Notificiations - Frequently Asked Questions v2.1'. https://covid19-static.cdn-apple.com/applications/covid19/current/static/contact-tracing/pdf/ExposureNotification-FAQv1.2.pdf.

Aristotle, and Jonathan Barnes. 2004. *The Nicomachean Ethics*. Edited by Hugh Tredennick. Translated by J. A. K. Thomson. New Ed edition. London, Eng.; New York, N.Y: Penguin Classics.

Beier, J. Marshall. 2003. 'Discriminating Tastes: "Smart" Bombs, Non-Combatants, and Notions of Legitimacy in Warfare'. *Security Dialogue* 34 (4): 411–25. https://doi.org/10.1177/0967010603344003.

Beier, J Marshall. 2006. 'Outsmarting Technologies: Rhetoric, Revolutions in Military Affairs, and the Social Depth of Warfare'. *International Politics* 43 (2): 266–80. https://doi.org/10.1057/palgrave.ip.8800144.

Bellaby, Ross W. 2014. *The Ethics of Intelligence: A New Framework*. London; New York: Routledge.

Burgess, Matt. 2020. 'Coronavirus Contact Tracing Apps Were Meant to Save Us. They Won't'. *Wired UK*, 30 April 2020. https://www.wired.co.uk/article/contact-tracing-apps-coronavirus.

Cappelen, Alexander W., and Bertil Tungodden. 2017. 'Fairness and the Proportionality Principle'. *Social Choice and Welfare* 49 (3–4): 709–19. https://doi.org/10.1007/s00355-016-1016-6.

Cavanaugh, T. A. 2006. *Double-Effect Reasoning: Doing Good and Avoiding Evil*. Oxford Studies in Theological Ethics. Oxford: Clarendon Press.

Cheyne, Ilona, and John Alder. 2007. 'Environmental Ethics and Proportionality: Hunting for a Balance'. *Environmental Law Review* 9 (3): 171–89. https://doi.org/10.1350/enlr.2007.9.3.171.

De Hert, Paul. 2005. 'Balancing Security and Liberty within the European Human Rights Framework. A Critical Reading of the Court's Case Law in the Light of Surveillance and Criminal Law Enforcement Strategies after 9/11 Special Issue on Terrorism'. *Utrecht Law Review* 1 (1): 68–96.

De La Garza, Alejandro. 2020. 'Why Aren't Contact Tracing Apps Working?' Time. 10 November 2020. https://time.com/5905772/covid-19-contact-tracing-apps/.

Esposito, C., A. De Santis, G. Tortora, H. Chang, and K. R. Choo. 2018. 'Blockchain: A Panacea for Healthcare Cloud-Based Data Security and Privacy?' *IEEE Cloud Computing* 5 (1): 31–37. https://doi.org/10.1109/MCC.2018.011791712.

Field, Matthew. 2020. 'No "real-World Evidence" That Contact Tracing Apps Work, Research Claims'. *The Telegraph*, 19 August 2020. https://www.telegraph.co.uk/technology/2020/08/19/no-real-world-evidence-contact-tracing-apps-work-research-claims/.

Fraser, Christophe, Lucie Abeler-Dorner, Luca Feretti, Michael Parker, Michelle Kendall, and David Bonsall. 2020. 'Digital Contact Tracing: Comparing the Capabilities of Centralised and Decentralised Data Architectures to Effectively Suppress the COVID-19 Epidemic Whilst Maximising Freedom of Movement and Maintaining Privacy'. GitHub. 7 May 2020. https://github.com/BDI-pathogens/covid-19_instant_tracing.

Gazendam, H. W. M, and A. H. M Kerkhoff. 1999. 'Information Technology: A Panacea?'

Henschke, Adam. 2018. 'Are The Costs Of Metadata Worth It? Conceptualising Proportionality And Its Relation To Metadata'. In *Intelligence and the Function of Government*, edited by Daniel Baldino and Rhys Crawley. Melbourne University Press.

Huesemann, Michael, and Joyce Huesemann. 2011. *Techno-Fix: Why Technology Won't Save Us Or the Environment*. New Society Publishers.

Hurka, Thomas. 2005. 'Proportionality in the Morality of War'. *Philosophy and Public Affairs* 33 (1): 34–66.

Iachello, Giovanni, and Gregory D. Abowd. 2005. 'Privacy and Proportionality: Adapting Legal Evaluation Techniques to Inform Design in Ubiquitous Computing'. In *Proceedings of the SIGCHI Conference on Human Factors in Computing Systems*, 91–100. CHI '05. New York, NY, USA: ACM. https://doi.org/10.1145/1054972.1054986.

IPA. 2016. *Investigatory Powers Act*. http://www.legislation.gov.uk/ukpga/2016/25/contents/enacted.

Johnston, Sean F. 2020. *Techno-Fixers: Origins and Implications of Technological Faith*. McGill-Queen's Press - MQUP.

Kamm, Frances M. 1991. 'The Doctrine of Double Effect: Reflections on Theoretical and Practical Issues'. *Journal of Medicine and Philosophy* 16 (5): 571–85. https://doi.org/10.1093/jmp/16.5.571.

Kim, Nemo. 2020. 'South Korea Struggles to Contain New Outbreak amid Anti-Gay Backlash'. *The Guardian*, 11 May 2020, sec. World news. https://www.theguardian.com/world/2020/may/11/south-korea-struggles-to-contain-new-outbreak-amid-anti-lgbt-backlash.

Klar, Renate, and Dirk Lanzerath. 2020. 'The Ethics of COVID-19 Tracking Apps– Challenges and Voluntariness'. *Research Ethics* 16 (3–4): 1–9.

Koptyug, Evgeniya. 2021. 'Coronavirus (COVID-19) Tracing App Downloads Germany 2020'. Statista. 18 January 2021. https://www.statista.com/statistics/1127547/coronavirus-covid-19-tracing-app-downloads-by-os-germany/.

Kostka, Genia, and Sabrina Habich-Sobiegalla. 2020. 'In Times of Crisis: Public Perceptions Towards COVID-19 Contact Tracing Apps in China, Germany and the US'. SSRN Scholarly Paper ID 3693783. Rochester, NY: Social Science Research Network. https://doi.org/10.2139/ssrn.3693783.

Krommendijk, Jasper, and John Morijn. 2009. '"Proportional" by What Measure(s)? Balancing Investor Interests and Human Rights by Way of Applying the Proportionality Principle in Investor-State Arbitration'. In *Human Rights in International Investment Law and Arbitration*, edited by Pierre-Marie Dupuy, Ernst-Ulrich Petersmann, and Francesco Francioni, 421–55. Oxford: Oxford University Press. https://papers.ssrn.com/abstract=2333550.

Li, Jinfeng, and Xinyi Guo. 2020. 'COVID-19 Contact-Tracing Apps: A Survey on the Global Deployment and Challenges'. *ArXiv:2005.03599 [Cs]*, May. http://arxiv.org/abs/2005.03599.

Macnish, Kevin. 2014. 'Just Surveillance? Towards a Normative Theory of Surveillance'. *Surveillance and Society* 12 (1): 142–53.

Macnish, Kevin. 2015. 'An Eye for an Eye: Proportionality and Surveillance'. *Ethical Theory and Moral Practice* 18 (3): 529–48. https://doi.org/10.1007/s10677-014-9537-5.

Macnish, Kevin. 2018. *The Ethics of Surveillance: An Introduction*. 1 edition. London : New York: Routledge.

Mcmahan, Jeff. 2011. *Killing in War*. Reprint edition. New York: Oxford University Press, U.S.A.

Michaelsen, Christopher. 2010. 'The Proportionality Principle, Counter-Terrorism Laws and Human Rights: A German-Australian Comparison'. *City University of Hong Kong Law Review* 2 (1): 19–44.

Nissenbaum, Helen. 2011. 'A Contextual Approach to Privacy Online'. *Daedalus* 140 (4): 32–48. https://doi.org/10.1162/DAED_a_00113.

Omand, David. 2012. *Securing the State*. London: Hurst.

Pagliari, Claudia. 2020. 'The Ethics and Value of Contact Tracing Apps: International Insights and Implications for Scotland's COVID-19 Response'. *Journal of Global Health* 10 (2). https://doi.org/10.7189/jogh.10.020103.

Pomarède, Julien. 2018. 'Normalizing Violence through Front-Line Stories: The Case of American Sniper'. *Critical Military Studies* 4 (1): 52–71. https://doi.org/10.1080/23337486.2016.1246995.

Quinlan, Michael. 2007. 'Just Intelligence: Prolegomena to an Ethical Theory'. *Intelligence and National Security* 22 (1): 1–13.

Quinn, Warren S. 1989. 'Actions, Intentions, and Consequences: The Doctrine of Double Effect'. *Philosophy and Public Affairs* 18 (4): 334–51.

Raman, Raghu, Krishnashree Achuthan, Ricardo Vinuesa, and Prema Nedungadi. 2021. 'COVIDTAS - COVID Tracing App Scale - an Evaluation Framework'. *Sustainability*.

Reuters. 2020. 'French COVID Tracing App Needs More Downloads to Be Effective: Minister'. *Reuters*, 25 October 2020. https://www.reuters.com/article/us-health-coronavirus-france-apps-idUSKBN27A0AZ.

Rønn, Kira Vrist, and Kasper Lippert-Rasmussen. 2020. 'Out of Proportion? On Surveillance and the Proportionality Requirement'. *Ethical Theory and Moral Practice*, 1–19.

Ryan, Mark. 2020. 'In Defence of Digital Contact-Tracing: Human Rights, South Korea and Covid-19'. *International Journal of Pervasive Computing and Communications* 16 (4): 383–407. https://doi.org/10.1108/IJPCC-07-2020-0081.

Sato, Mia. 2020. 'Contact Tracing Apps Now Cover Nearly Half of America. It's Not Too Late to Use One.' MIT Technology Review. 14 December 2020. https://www.technologyreview.com/2020/12/14/1014426/covid-california-contact-tracing-app-america-states/.

Sharon, Tamar. 2020. 'Blind-Sided by Privacy? Digital Contact Tracing, the Apple/Google API and Big Tech's Newfound Role as Global Health Policy Makers'. *Ethics and Information Technology*, July. https://doi.org/10.1007/s10676-020-09547-x.

Singh, Deepti, and Daniel Thomas. 2019. 'Advances in Medical Polymer Technology towards the Panacea of Complex 3D Tissue and Organ Manufacture'. *The American Journal of Surgery* 217 (4): 807–8. https://doi.org/10.1016/j.amjsurg.2018.05.012.

Slobogin, Christopher. 1998. 'Let's Not Bury Terry: A Call for Rejuvenation of the Proportionality Principle'...*John's L. Rev.* 72: 1053.

Steel, Daniel. 2013. 'Precaution and Proportionality: A Reply to Turner'. *Ethics, Policy & Environment* 16 (3): 344–48. https://doi.org/10.1080/21550085.2013.844572.

Tapper, James. 2020. 'Minorities More at Risk from Covid-19 Because of Racism, Says Report'. *The Guardian*, 13 June 2020, sec. Inequality. http://www.theguardian.com/inequality/2020/jun/13/leaked-report-says-racism-and-inequality-increase-covid-19-risk-for-minorities.

Thomsen, Frej Klem. 2020. 'The Teleological Account of Proportional Surveillance'. *Res Publica*, 1–29.

Tierney, Thomas F. 1992. *The Value of Convenience: A Genealogy of Technical Culture*. Albany: State University of New York Press.

Turner, Derek. 2013. 'Proportionality and the Precautionary Principle'. *Ethics, Policy & Environment* 16 (3): 341–43. https://doi.org/10.1080/21550085.2013.844571.

Uniacke, Suzanne. 2011. 'Proportionality and Self-Defense'. *Law and Philosophy* 30 (3): 253–72.

Wells, Helen. 2008. 'The Techno-Fix Versus The Fair Cop: Procedural (In)Justice and Automated Speed Limit Enforcement'. *The British Journal of Criminology* 48 (6): 798–817. https://doi.org/10.1093/bjc/azn058.

Williams, R. D. 2001. 'Is the West's Reliance on Technology the Panacea for Future Conflict or Its Achilles' Heel?' *Defence Studies* 1 (2): 38–56. https://doi.org/10.1080/714000026.

Williams, Simon N., Christopher J. Armitage, Tova Tampe, and Kimberly Dienes. 2021. 'Public Attitudes towards COVID-19 Contact Tracing Apps: A UK-Based Focus Group Study'. *Health Expectations* n/a (n/a). https://doi.org/10.1111/hex.13179.

# Index

Denmark 105
Deontology 30–1, 42, 190, 196
Dictatorship 5, 31–2, 36–41
Digital Divide 3
Digital literacy 181
Discrimination 52, 61–2, 66–72, 77, 137
Discrimination, principle of 98, 191–92, 203
Distribution of information 9, 170, 179
Distribution of risk 63–8, 104, 113, 124, 127, 129, 161, 194–95, 210
Domination 5, 26, 31–44

Ebola 116, 174, 192
Election 34, 41, 169
Epidemiology 4, 26–7, 60, 112, 115, 117, 125, 127
Epistemic injustice 6, 76–7, 84–88
Ethics by design 8, 167f
Ethics of Care, see also Care
Exception* 30, 52, 83–4, 133, 150, 161–62, 186–99
Extinction Rebellion 132–33

Fairness 55, 61–2, 65, 72, 76, 86, 113, 127, 129, 156, 157, 198
False negatives 9, 204, 208
False positives 9, 119, 204, 208
Floridi, Luciano 70, 72
France 209
Freedom 1, 4, 6, 19, 25, 32–4, 41–4, 95, 100, 134–35, 137, 143, 145, 153–56, 169, 209
Function creep 2, 4–9, 50, 52, 160

GCHQ 4, 15
General Data Protection Regulation (GDPR) 61, 67–9
Germany 209
Gonorrhoea 116
Google 22, 54, 80–1, 111, 116, 203, 206–09
GPS 6, 21, 50, 58, 60, 66, 113, 206

Habeas corpus 30, 40–41
Haiti 60
Healthcare 1, 20, 56, 76–83, 103, 112, 118, 127–28, 159, 198, 206, 208, 210
HIV 116

Identify 2, 3, 7, 16, 18, 21, 25, 52, 81, 103, 111, 114, 116, 136, 151–52, 176–77, 210–11
Identity 49, 68–72, 77, 85, 152
Immunity 37, 43
Infiltration 136, 140–46
Information, personal 2, 6, 7, 17, 49, 51, 61, 68–70, 80, 103, 105, 111, 116, 122, 127, 206–07

Information, private 2, 17–19, 21, 51, 61, 65–67, 72, 104, 113, 115, 141, 152, 176, 198
Information, public 52, 60, 77, 152
Injustice, hermeneutical 84
Injustice, testimonial 76, 84–7
Interference 26, 33, 124, 142, 145, 154
iOS 49
Isolation 4, 19, 23, 27, 30, 96, 101–05, 122, 127, 153, 208, 210, 212
Israel 49, 121, 151, 153

Japan 17, 171
Justice, procedural 31, 40–42, 157

Liability 6–7, 15, 41–4, 66, 95–103, 106–08, 120, 192
Libertarianism 27, 157
Liberty 4, 38, 44, 111, 124, 136, 154, 157, 173–74
Lockdown 1, 16–7, 20, 22, 32, 43, 47, 52–3, 85, 112, 118–19, 122, 127, 132, 152, 155, 157

Machiavelli 36–7
Malaria 60
McMahan, Jeff 97–8, 100–01
Merkel, Angela 26
MERS 116
Metadata 5, 24–5, 47–52, 57–8, 68
Mill, John Stuart 123, 209
Mission creep 65
Mobile phone* 3, 5–6, 17–18, 20–22, 47–9, 54, 56–7, 60, 66, 85, 96, 100, 113, 116, 119, 121–22, 186, 207
Morley, Jessica 170–80

National Health Service (UK) 20–3, 117
National Security Agency (US) 4, 15, 24–6
Natural disasters 191
Nazi experiments 64, 82
Negligence 101–07
NHS, see National Health Service (UK)
Norway 50
Nozick, Robert 99–101
NSA, see National Security Agency (US)

Orwell, George 27
Ottawa 155

Pandemic 1–9, 15–27, 30, 35, 41, 43–4, 47–54, 57–58, 61, 65–7, 76–77, 80, 83, 95–6, 105, 108, 111–12, 116–20, 122, 125–26, 128–29, 132, 134, 146, 150–63, 169–83, 186–89, 191–94, 198, 209, 212
Paternalism 97, 107–08